Bion and Psychosis

This comprehensive work systematically describes Wilfred Bion's work on psychosis and critically develops his contribution in order to arrive at an appropriate and modern understanding of the disorder.

The book provides deep insights into the psychoanalytic treatment of psychotic patients through comprehensive analysis of key concepts including the alpha function, the failure to dream, and psychic retreat. It bridges theoretical understanding with clinical application, examining how psychotic minds function as sensory organs rather than thinking apparatus, and offers practical guidance for therapeutic work with severely impacted patients. The text critically evaluates both the achievements and limitations of Kleinian approaches while presenting fresh perspectives on childhood withdrawal and delusional structure formation.

Bion and Psychosis is essential reading for psychoanalysts, psychiatrists, clinical psychologists, and mental health professionals working with psychotic patients. It serves as an invaluable resource for trainees, postgraduate students and researchers in psychoanalysis, particularly those studying Kleinian theory, Bion's work, or severe mental disorders.

Franco De Masi is a training and supervising analyst based in Milan, Italy. He is the author of *Psychosis: A Contemporary Introduction* (2026) and *A Psychoanalytic Approach to Treating Psychosis* (2020).

The Routledge Wilfred R. Bion Studies Book Series

Series Editor
Howard B. Levine, MD

The contributions of Wilfred Bion are among the most cited in the analytic literature. Their appeal lies not only in their content and explanatory value, but in their generative potential. Although Bion's training and many of his clinical instincts were deeply rooted in the classical tradition of Melanie Klein, his ideas have a potentially universal appeal. Rather than emphasizing a particular psychic content (e.g., Oedipal conflicts in need of resolution; splits that needed to be healed; preconceived transferences that must be allowed to form and flourish, etc.), he tried to help open and prepare the mind of the analyst (without memory, desire or theoretical preconception) for the encounter with the patient.

Bion's formulations of group mentality and the psychotic and non-psychotic portions of the mind, his theory of thinking and emphasis on facing and articulating the truth of one's existence so that one might truly learn firsthand from one's own experience, his description of psychic development (alpha function and container/contained) and his exploration of O are "non-denominational" concepts that defy relegation to a particular school or orientation of psychoanalysis. Consequently, his ideas have taken root in many places… and those ideas continue to inform many different branches of psychoanalytic inquiry and interest.[1]

It is with this heritage and its promise for the future developments of psychoanalysis in mind that we present *The Routledge Wilfred Bion Studies Book Series.* This series gathers together newly emerging and continually evolving contributions to psychoanalytic thinking that rest upon Bion's foundational texts and explore and extend the implications of his thought. For a full list of titles in the series, please visit the Routledge website at: https://www.routledge.com/The-Routledge-Wilfred-Bion-Studies-Book-Series/book-series/RWBSBS

Howard B. Levine, MD
Series Editor

1 Levine, H.B. and Civitarese, G. (2016). Editors' Preface, *The W.R. Bion Tradition*, Levine and Civitarese, eds., London: Karnac 2016, p. xxi.

Bion and Psychosis

A Long Road to Clinical Discovery

Franco De Masi

Routledge
Taylor & Francis Group
LONDON AND NEW YORK

Designed cover image: *Return from the Wood*, 1890 by Giovanni Segantini

First published 2027
by Routledge
4 Park Square, Milton Park, Abingdon, Oxon OX14 4RN

and by Routledge
605 Third Avenue, New York, NY 10158

Routledge is an imprint of the Taylor & Francis Group, an informa business

Translated by Olivia Melani

British Library Cataloguing in Publication Data
A catalogue record for this book is available from the British Library

ISBN: 978-1-041-28580-9 (hbk)
ISBN: 978-1-041-28578-6 (pbk)
ISBN: 978-1-003-76536-3 (ebk)

DOI: 10.4324/9781003765363

Typeset in Times New Roman
by Taylor & Francis Books

Contents

Premise

This book has been conceived with a plurality of aims. Above all, it seeks to retrace Bion's trajectory in his exploration of psychosis, elucidating the originality of his contributions while interrogating the conceptual premises from which his work emerged. My central hypothesis is that, although Bion opened unforeseen perspectives in the study of the human mind and offered extraordinary insights into psychotic functioning, he did not arrive at a definitive or exhaustive understanding of the disorder.

The conjunction contained in the title, *Bion and Psychosis*, should therefore also be read in a disjunctive sense. On the one hand, there is Bion, with the richness of his thought and his reflections on psychosis; on the other, there is psychosis itself, a psychic reality that still demands further investigation if it is to be comprehended in its full scope and complexity. From this perspective, I offer a number of considerations matured over decades of study and clinical practice, concerning the origins and development of the psychotic process.

With Bion, the psyche assumed a dynamic and transformative quality that no previous theoretical framework had ever attributed to it. His intuitions regarding the nature of thought and dreaming, the transformations of psychic elements, the creative function of the unconscious, and the distinction between neurotic and psychotic structures opened up an unprecedented horizon for the understanding of psychosis.

The first part of the present volume is devoted to the formative stages of Bion's thinking on psychosis and, in particular, to an analysis of *Second Thoughts*, which collects his early writings. My aim will be to reconstruct the theoretical premises from which his inquiry originated and to highlight the clinical encounters that decisively shaped his reflections.

Bion's ideas frequently manifest themselves as sudden illuminations: they break through like flashes of lightning, casting a powerful light, while at the same time arousing a certain sense of awe. My intention, however, is to move beyond the immediate and dazzling quality of these insights, tracing the deeper roots of his thought and integrating the sometimes oracular, almost *ipse dixit*, register that not infrequently characterizes his writings.

Revisiting Bion's clinical writings on psychosis, one often has the impression that his interpretations descend from above: they appear to be generated more by the theoretical framework he has in mind at that moment than by the patient's associative flow or direct feedback. His intuitions emerge rapidly, almost like flashes of lightning; they arise from a gesture, a glance, or a patient's silence, which for Bion became signs of the ceaseless projective transformations taking place.

It should be recalled, however, that Bion was not alone, in those years, in working with psychotic patients and employing such a direct interpretative method. At his side were other members of the Kleinian group, among them Hanna Segal and Herbert Rosenfeld. Segal proceeded with greater caution and methodological care, leaving us with accounts of treatments conducted with a certain degree of success. Her patients, however, were not as severely psychotic as those encountered by Bion and Rosenfeld. The latter worked with subjects in acute phases or with chronic patients, at a time when no pharmacological means were yet available to support the most critical moments of the illness.

Bion and Rosenfeld moved forward with great confidence, convinced that they were opening a new path for psychoanalysis. In the wake of Melanie Klein's 1946 formulations, they believed they had found the key to penetrating the mystery of psychosis.

Yet, as I shall attempt to demonstrate in these pages, the hopes generated by those hypotheses progressively revealed themselves to be partial: insufficient both to disclose the true nature of the process and to outline a clinically viable model of treatment. Psychosis has, in fact, continued to present itself as an impregnable fortress, one that even today requires new tools for it to be adequately approached and understood.

Introduction

Psychosis remains, without doubt, the *black continent* of medicine, psychiatry, and psychoanalysis. Freud was among the first to attempt an exploration of its boundaries, through his commentary on the illness of President Schreber. In order to comprehend it, he applied the same method he had employed with neuroses: reading the patient's words as revelations of repressed unconscious conflicts. He thus arrived at the conclusion that Schreber's delusion had its origin in his repressed homosexuality.

In the years that followed, however, Freud acknowledged that psychoanalysis was engaged in an unequal struggle against psychosis. He declared that one would have to wait for more favorable times in order to hope to fully grasp the nature of this illness. He therefore placed his hopes in the future insights of his students and colleagues. The analytic method, to be sure, was not without its usefulness; yet it was evident that new horizons would be required, openings still difficult to envisage.

Towards the end of his life he wrote: "Thus we discover that we must renounce the idea of trying our treatment plan on psychotics—renounce it perhaps forever or perhaps only for the time being, till we have found some other plan better adapted for them" (Freud, 1938, vol. 23, p. 173).

A second phase in the analytic investigation of psychosis was inaugurated by Melanie Klein. In her view, the early infantile anxieties and fantasies of the primitive ego, together with its relation to its objects, allowed for the identification of the roots of this illness. The schizoparanoid position—alongside defenses such as splitting, fragmentation, and confusion—was not merely an archaic modality through which the infant related to objects, but also constituted the very nucleus of psychosis itself.

From this perspective, psychosis appears as the outcome of a primitive organization of the mind. The psyche of the psychotic patient, in fact, remains fixed at the schizoparanoid position, dominated by a rigid separation between the good and the bad. For this reason, the patient is unable to reach the depressive position, that psychic space in which positive and negative aspects can be integrated within the same object, opening the way to a more adequate vision of psychic reality.

DOI: 10.4324/9781003765363-1

The analogy drawn by Melanie Klein between the primitive and the pathological in psychosis led her pupils—among them Bion and Rosenfeld—to consider the analytic treatment of psychotic patients possible, both in acute and chronic phases. They highlighted how specific pathogenic nuclei are operative in the psychotic process: the massive use of projective identification, the loss of symbolic function, attacks on the object, the fragmentation of perceptual functions, and the confusion between inner and outer worlds. Psychotic transference thus became an indispensable tool for accessing and analyzing such pathogenic manifestations.

The point of departure for Bion and Rosenfeld is the same: a theoretical and clinical terrain deeply rooted in Klein's legacy. From there, however, the two move along parallel tracks. Many of the ideas of one can be found in the other, yet their styles diverge profoundly. Rosenfeld works methodically, constructing a clinical framework that is solid and systematic. Bion, by contrast, seems propelled by a different force: his writing is animated by a creative movement that generates conceptual insights of extraordinary originality.

Although it is true that his early works emerged under Klein's direct influence, from the very first pages one perceives a thought seeking its own space. Bion begins with the concrete experience of the analytic session, but his mind immediately pushes beyond it, toward broader truths capable of rising above the clinical datum. It is in this momentum that his most mature reflections take shape—on the functioning of the mind, on the meaning of dream and of the unconscious, on the distinction between neurotic and psychotic structures. These reflections retain, even today, their full vitality.

And yet, while these intuitions remain alive, the clinical path he outlined for the treatment of psychoses proves far more difficult to traverse. His hypotheses, born in a creative whirlwind, preserve their fascination and relevance, but rarely offer tools that can be immediately applied in analytic practice.

It is precisely from this impasse that the second part of the present work begins. I intend to propose some possible directions for the therapy of psychosis, inspired by the richness of Bion's insights yet moving from a different genetic perspective, one that does not place at the center the destructive processes of the psychotic mind. My aim will be to show, in the following pages, what is illuminating in the path opened by Bion and, at the same time, what still remains to be explored, developed, and integrated—so as to bring that legacy of thought closer to the needs of contemporary clinical practice.

Chapter 1

Antecedents

The psychoanalysts of the Kleinian group were among the first to develop a shared and coherent genetic theoretical vision of psychosis. To understand the origins of this collective convergence, it is necessary to return to Melanie Klein's seminal paper "Notes on Some Schizoid Mechanisms" (1946). That text became a kind of cornerstone, a stable foundation for all those within the group who engaged with the clinical and theoretical challenge posed by psychosis. I will therefore attempt to recall, in a synthetic way, the essential passages of that contribution.

Klein argued that the fixation points of psychosis are to be sought in the very earliest phases of life, when sadistic–oral impulses arouse persecutory fears that may constitute the original nucleus of future paranoia and schizophrenia.

A central element of her thinking is the emphasis placed on the action of the destructive drive, conceived as primary and endowed with a force so intense as to threaten the ego still in its formative state.

Under this pressure, the primitive ego tends to fragment—a movement Klein compared to what occurs in schizophrenic states of disintegration: "I suggest that the primary anxiety of being annihilated by a destructive force within, with the ego's specific response of falling to pieces or splitting itself, may be extremely important in all schizophrenic processes" (Klein, 1946, p. 5).

Alongside the destructive drive, Klein identified other mechanisms of the primitive ego that contribute to facilitating the development of psychotic disturbance. Among these, a significant role is played by the denial of psychic reality, which finds its roots in the feelings of omnipotence typical of the ego's earliest functioning.

It is precisely at this point that Melanie Klein introduces, for the first time, a concept destined to become central in psychoanalysis: *projective identification*.

She described it as the prototype of aggressive object relations, a psychic movement in which parts of the ego are evacuated and deposited into the object, giving rise to dynamics of control, intrusion, and attack—dynamics that would deeply shape the psychoanalytic understanding of psychoses:

DOI: 10.4324/9781003765363-2

> When projection is mainly derived from the infant's impulse to harm or to control the mother, he feels her to be a persecutor. In psychotic disorders this identification of an object with the hated parts of the self contributes to the intensity of the hatred directed against other people.
>
> (Klein, 1946, p. 8)

Klein underlines that the processes of splitting off parts of the self and projecting them into objects are thus of vital importance for normal development as well as for abnormal object relations.

She also says:

> If states of splitting and therefore of disintegration, which the ego is unable to overcome, occur too frequently and go on for too long, then in my view they must be regarded as a sign of schizophrenic illness in the infant, and some indications of such illness may already be seen in the first few months of life. In adult patients, states of depersonalization and of schizophrenic dissociation seem to be a regression to these infantile states of disintegration.
>
> (Klein, 1946, p. 10)

The perception that one's body or psyche is being controlled in a hostile manner by others expresses, for Klein, a profound distortion of the process of introjecting good objects. This distortion gives rise to a flight into the idealized object, as observed in psychotic states, where the ego seeks refuge in an internal image that offers protection against persecutory threats.

In describing the transition from the schizoparanoid position to the depressive one—which constitutes the normal developmental passage of the mind—Klein notes that when persecutory anxieties and the corresponding schizoid mechanisms are excessively intense, the ego proves unable to work through the depressive position. In such cases, it is compelled to regress repeatedly to the schizoparanoid position, thereby reinforcing persecutory anxieties rather than transforming them. In this way, the evolutionary process that would normally lead to greater integration of emotional experience is interrupted, leading to a split and fragmented mode of functioning.

According to Klein, this dynamic creates the basis upon which various forms of adult schizophrenia may take root: the mind becomes trapped within a defensive circuit that obstructs integration and prevents the psychic work demanded by loss and ambivalence.

Klein's theory thus provides a powerful interpretive key for understanding how the roots of adult psychoses are anchored in the earliest stages of psychic life, when the ego—fragile and besieged by destructive drives—desperately attempts to defend itself through mechanisms that ultimately serve to entrap it.

In summary, Melanie Klein situates the origins of psychosis within the very first months of life, at the point where normal developmental processes may come to a halt. Under such circumstances, the mental organization remains dominated by psychic configurations which, if excessively persistent in adulthood, take on a pathological character.

Among the mechanisms involved, particular significance is attributed to the splitting of internal and external objects, of affectivity, and of the ego itself. These operations are part of normal development, yet when they become rigidified they form the nucleus of future schizophrenic conditions.

A central role is also assigned to projective identification—a combination of splitting and projection of parts of the self onto others. It is precisely this dynamic that produces the confusion of identities and leaves a deep imprint on the structure of the psychotic mind.

The Primitive and the Pathological

Through this conceptualization, Klein resumes a line of thought several analytic theories have referred to: pathology is identified with the primitive and the unevolved. What produces pathology is nothing other than the predominance of primitive and pathological modes of mental functioning.

According to this hypothesis, psychosis does not emerge from a distorted developmental trajectory absent in normal growth, but rather belongs to the primitive organization of the psyche itself.

In other words, Klein establishes an analogy between advanced psychotic symptomatology—in which dissociative and projective mechanisms prevail—and the functioning of the primitive mind, which operates according to the same principle.

It should be noted, then, that Klein's model places the late manifestations of psychosis—such as dissociation or persecutory anxiety—in direct continuity with the structure of the primitive ego. In this way, the process is inscribed within a self-enclosed, circular system, one that makes it difficult to introduce additional elements of understanding.

From this perspective, the origins of illness appear predetermined, and the clinical approach becomes inevitably conditioned by this presupposition. The risk is that manifestations which could be understood as late expressions of illness—such as dissociation, fragmentation of the ego, extreme projective identification, and hallucinatory phenomena—may instead be regarded as primitive in themselves.

As we shall see in the following pages, both Bion and Rosenfeld—at least in an initial phase—pursued this path, with the attendant risk of finding themselves in a theoretical and clinical dead end. Both, however, were later compelled to broaden their horizons of inquiry: Bion through his luminous insights into the theory of thinking, and Rosenfeld by reconsidering, with increasing rigor, the clinical perspective from which he had originally set out.

Within Klein's model, a central role is assigned to the destructive drive, regarded as the primary force capable of producing the disintegration that characterizes psychotic transformation. It is around this destructive energy that Klein builds much of her understanding of psychosis: it threatens the primitive ego, compels it to fragment, and generates mechanisms—splitting, projection, projective identification—that constitute the matrix of future schizophrenic disturbances.

Melanie Klein conceived anxiety as the result of the death instinct going into operation and being perceived as fear of annihilation; this destructive instinct is projected onto an object that becomes omnipotent, uncontrollable, and persecuting. Anxiety connected to being annihilated by an inner destructive force results in the fragmentation and splitting of the Ego: the more sadism predominates in introjection, the greater the fragmentation of the incorporated object, the Ego splitting correspondingly.

Another important process is object idealization, which, on the one hand, defends from persecution, but on the other, expresses the omnipotent desire to have a breast infinitely on hand. This process occurs in the infantile hallucinatory world and in psychosis and is created by virtue of the splitting of the object, denial of frustration, and persecution. All this leads to psychic reality being blotted out. In this early stage, splitting, denial, and omnipotence perform a function analogous to that of repression in more advanced stages of development.

Melanie Klein claimed that these infantile world primitive modalities are reproduced in psychosis, and here she connects back to Freud and his assertion (1924b) that, whereas in neurosis "the loss" follows repression, in psychosis the more radical mechanism of "disavowal" is in operation. It is not the drive that is repressed in psychosis but the perception of external reality.

In particular, when projective identification is massive it becomes difficult to take back possession of the projected parts. When emotions and parts of the self are alienated and placed in other people, besides confusion between self and object, emotional voids form in the patient's inner world. The feeling of psychic death experienced by psychotic patients derives from the loss of important parts of the self and from the evacuation of the emotional world.

This is the conceptual framework to which Kleinian analysts—such as Bion, Rosenfeld, and Segal—referred in their work with psychosis. In particular, attention was directed to the patient's use of projective identification, regarded as one of the principal avenues for interpretive work.

Identity Change

In her 1955 paper "On Identification," Klein significantly broadened the scope of this concept, demonstrating how it illuminates the patient's loss of identity in psychosis.

On the basis of a story by Julien Green (1947), Klein tells how Fabien, who is depressed and unhappy, makes a pact with the devil to enable him to transform himself into a different person. Before changing into his college president, a wealthy and seemingly happy old man, Fabien notes down the address of the house where he lives with his mother. He is worried at the possibility of total loss of his former identity, and of not being able to go back.

Having transformed himself into the college president, he notices that he has acquired not only the desirable but also the negative characteristics of this person: he has become an old man. So he decides to exchange identities with an athletic youngster he meets in a bar, but always takes the precaution of slipping the address into his pocket before effecting the transformation.

As he progressively enters into other admired and envied characters, Fabien realizes that he is increasingly losing the perception of his original identity, and becomes aware of the risk of finding himself permanently trapped in one of the persons into whom he has penetrated. This perception arouses anxiety when he discovers that the last young man whose identity he has assumed is a murderer who has killed his female partner.

To avoid being arrested, he again becomes a different person, but begins to feel more and more uncomfortable and acutely claustrophobic. In order to recover his own lost identity, he must embark on a backward odyssey, returning in reverse order through the characters with whom he has exchanged identities. After a difficult experience of reconquest and integration of his self, in the end he recognizes his house, where he comes to from a faint, watched over by the mother from whom he has never separated.

Through the vicissitudes of Fabien, Melanie Klein describes the transformations of identity that take place in psychosis and their underlying mechanisms. The prime mover is envy of the admired qualities of the object and the wish to appropriate them for oneself in fantasy. The projection of parts of the self into the object impoverishes the personality, which may even be totally lost.

Despite its varied clinical manifestations, projective identification remains a central concept for the understanding of psychotic psychopathology. It makes it possible to discern the profound alteration of identity that takes place in the course of the pathological process, when split-off parts of the self are evacuated and deposited into the object, thereby producing identity confusion, distortions, and intrusions that mark the patient's psychic life.

As I shall argue later, it seems to me that the notion of projective identification as described by Klein represents only one aspect of a more complex phenomenon of transformation. In the psychotic process, projective identification—that is, the transformation of identity—does not always occur with real objects, even if idealized or envied, but rather with omnipotent figures created by fantasy, rooted in a megalomaniac world in which the patient is immersed.

Among those who, alongside Bion, most faithfully followed Melanie Klein's theoretical indications and translated them into the clinical domain was undoubtedly Herbert Rosenfeld.

One of the concepts that inspired his work was that psychotic illness originates from aggressive fantasies and persecutory anxieties rooted in early childhood, to the point that the psychotic patient remains imprisoned within his illness because of an excess of primary sadism. In his volume *Psychotic States* (Rosenfeld, 1965), he described how it was possible to treat both acute and chronic patients through the use of psychoanalytic technique.

Psychotic Transference

Rosenfeld's underlying hypothesis is that the psychoanalytic method, grounded in the analysis of transference, could be employed in the treatment of psychosis without resorting to reassurance or educational measures:

> It has been found that the psychotic manifestations attach themselves to the transference in both acute and chronic conditions, so that what one may call a "transference psychosis" develops. The analyst's main task in both acute and chronic schizophrenias is the recognition of the relevant transference phenomena and its communication to the patient.
>
> (1965, p. 117)

Rosenfeld believed that schizophrenic patients concretely experienced the sensation of entering into the analyst at the beginning of the session through projective identification, only to feel expelled at the end. Splitting and projective identification, at work in the psychotic state, thus account for the patient's lack of sense of identity, the loss of affects, and the difficulty in the use of symbols.

Despite this gravely impaired level of functioning and the disturbance of symbolic capacity brought about by excessive projective identification, Rosenfeld maintained that it was nevertheless useful to resort to interpretation: interpreting projective identification, in fact, tended to facilitate the patient's understanding of the analyst's communications.

Rosenfeld consistently interpreted the fragmented, anguished, and persecutory state in relation to the transference, highlighting the dynamics of projective identification; in particular, he emphasized the aggressive fantasies toward the analyst, the corresponding death threats emanating from the Superego, and the manifestations of primary envy.

In the face of Rosenfeld's tenacity—tireless in his effort to enter the world of his most severely psychotic patients—one is struck by an ambivalent sentiment. On the one hand, admiration for his clinical dedication; on the other, perplexity: how could those patients, torn apart by confusion and dissociation, truly comprehend and internally utilize the interpretations they received?

Rosenfeld, however, did not retreat in the face of this question. He believed that psychotic transference was a threshold rather than an obstacle: to interpret it meant to accompany the patient into the very heart of the delusion, into that place where the analyst was engulfed and confused with persecutory or salvific internal figures.

It was precisely at this point of fusion that he discerned a clinical benefit, going so far as to assert with determination: "The success of the analysis depends on our understanding of the psychotic manifestations in the transference situation" (1952, p. 65).

This position would later be abandoned (1987) when Rosenfeld stated that psychotic transference is dangerous, since in this case the delusion may engulf the figure of the analyst, thereby paralyzing his analytic function as a transformative object.

Chapter 2

Early Bion

To present Bion's work on psychosis, I will refer to *Second Thoughts* (1967), which gathers his writings from the 1950s and 1960s—papers originally presented at international congresses or to the British Psychoanalytical Society, later supplemented with retrospective commentary. The very title indicates a reflection undertaken *a posteriori*.

The most significant texts in this perspective are: "Notes on the Theory of Schizophrenia" (1954), "The Development of Schizophrenic Thought" (1956), "Differentiation of the Psychotic from the Non-Psychotic Personalities" (1957), "On Hallucination" (1958), and "Attacks on Linking" (1959).

In these works, unlike in his later period, Bion is in the analytic room with the patient: his elaborations arise directly from the immediate experience of the analytic encounter with psychotic patients. Only later will psychosis appear intermittently, as a useful dialectical counterpoint to his broader investigation into the nature and function of thought.

In the cases presented in these writings, the patients are situated in an active psychotic phase. Bion provides no details about their personal history, nor about the onset or development of the disorder; in fact, he does not even consider the mental state preceding the session. He confines himself to presenting the patient *in vivo*, within the analytic room, and describing what unfolds in the interactive dynamic with the analyst.

This choice is deliberate. Bion's interest does not lie in the patient's biography or personal identity, but in the functioning of the psychotic mind during the session, observed in its immediate impact with interpretation. What attracts him is the process itself, the way in which the patient reacts moment by moment to the analytic intervention, in a relationship that may at times take on the intensity of a veritable hand-to-hand struggle.

Since the psychotic patient is not capable of providing coherent verbal responses, Bion considers other forms of reaction: fragmentary exclamations, movements, aggressive attitudes. It is precisely in these signals that he identifies the index of an effective interpretation, one capable of intercepting the living core of psychotic communication.

DOI: 10.4324/9781003765363-3

In his early writings, a certain detachment from the patient is evident: the session appears almost as the testing ground for the solidity of his theoretical constructions. At that stage, the impression is that Bion, following in Klein's footsteps, believed himself to hold sufficient keys to unlock the mystery of psychosis.

Only later would his exploration expand toward a broader and more dynamic vision. The psychotic world is no longer enclosed within the rigid Kleinian axiom of destructiveness, but begins to be conceived as an originary lack: the absence of the function of thought and of the creative capacity of the unconscious.

This marks a significant turning point, although Bion—like Freud—never explicitly renounced his earlier hypotheses, even when they appear to contradict his new conceptualizations.

Thus, Klein's emphasis on the destructive drive as the fundamental feature of psychotic functioning persists, even when Bion, in the most transformative passages of the later phase of these early writings, seems able to situate psychosis within a more original matrix, defined by the function of thought and not solely by destructiveness.

"Notes on the Theory of Schizophrenia" (1954)

In this paper, projective identification—understood in its destructive form and aimed at disintegrating the object—assumes a central role, one that will remain a constant point in Bion's reflections for years. He observes how the indiscriminate use of this mechanism produces decisive consequences: the blockage of symbolic capacity, the fragmentation and distortion of language, and the splitting of the analyst into two opposing figures, one benevolent and the other persecutory.

The reference to Freud is explicit. In *Neurosis and Psychosis* (1924a), Freud distinguished neurosis as the outcome of a conflict between Ego and Id, whereas psychosis derives from a disturbance in the relation between Ego and external reality.

Hence, the two structures are not superimposable: in neurosis the nucleus is conflictual, whereas in psychosis one does not find an unconscious conflict in the strict sense, but rather a rupture with the external world.

Bion also recalls another Freudian text, *Formulations on the Two Principles of Mental Functioning* (1911), in which Freud noted that the sense organs, beyond transmitting pleasure and pain, progressively develop an additional function: the perception of meaning and the awareness of reality. It is precisely this function that is compromised in psychosis, giving way to a perceptual modality dominated by the attack on the object.

The patient, Bion observes, is unable to grasp the meaning of events, having never moved beyond a perceptual modality restricted to pleasure and pain. In his view, this developmental arrest derives from destructive attacks directed against the very maturation of the perceptual organs. The consequence is an incapacity to employ verbal thought, which presupposes the acquisition of the depressive position—the only psychic condition capable of integrating opposites and initiating a process of reparation.

Bion further underscores how the structural link between the depressive position and verbal thought helps explain the hatred that the psychotic patient harbors toward analysis. The analytic cure, in fact, is founded upon language and symbolic work—precisely that which the patient perceives as an intolerable threat to his psychic functioning.

Bion's technique rests directly on these theoretical premises. Psychosis is traced back to an early stage of development, dominated by destructive fantasies toward the primary object, the mother. If such fantasies are not transformed through reparative processes, pathological mental structures consolidate, predisposing the subject to the onset of illness. The destruction of reality renders reparation an exceedingly difficult task: through analytic work the patient may acquire some degree of awareness of psychic reality, yet remains unable to tolerate the acknowledgment of the destruction that has taken place.

In moments when the patient succeeds in thinking, he experiences a psychic pain so intense as to induce an immediate disinvestment of every capacity for understanding.

Thus, whenever he regains—even partially—an awareness of psychic reality, hatred toward the analyst becomes inevitable: the analyst is experienced as the one who has forced him to confront the catastrophe that has occurred. In those cases where progress is observed, Bion does not speak of cure but of an enhanced capacity for adaptation to reality—a partial improvement that does not eliminate the underlying pathology.

For Bion, the difficulty of emerging from the psychotic state lies in the impossibility of accessing the depressive position. Only this position would allow the integration of language and thought, otherwise compromised by the massive splittings that characterize psychotic experience.

The theme of the failure to achieve the depressive position recurs frequently in the writings of Klein's followers. The shared perspective was that fixation in a schizoparanoid position precluded symbolic elaboration and maintained the subject in a condition of fragmentation, deprived of the reparative possibilities proper to the depressive position.

Hanna Segal, for example, in "Depression in the Schizophrenic" (1956), claimed that the psychotic patient is unable to tolerate depressive anxiety and regresses when this looms large.

In one session, her patient had an insight and asked the analyst if by chance her problem happened to be that of constantly eating and taking things inside her without making any effort to build something good inside.

For Hanna Segal, this was the moment of depression. After this session, in which the patient seemed more pensive and mentally healthy, she arrived for her next session with a dissociated, masturbatory, and incoherent attitude, ignoring the analyst entirely.

Hanna Segal saw this behavior as a negative therapeutic reaction: experiencing being solely destructive and draining the breast had made the patient feel unable to repair and reconstruct it. Hanna Segal's conclusion was that, as long as the patient had been able to keep her depressive feelings inside her, she could communicate healthily; when these depressive feelings became unbearable, she needed to project them onto the analyst, resulting in a loss of reality, a return to mad behavior and the reappearance of persecutory feelings. In this case, the analyst had become the persecutor who contained the patient's depressive part, which she intended to push back into her.

A similar view was expressed by Rosenfeld, when he wrote:

> However, when aggressive impulses become temporarily predominant, the reparative process may be interfered with in particular way. The libidinal impulses succeed in bringing the pieces of the objects and the ego together, nevertheless the aggressive impulses prevent these pieces from being sorted out and put together correctly.
>
> (Rosenfeld, 1950, p. 137)

Bion, however, does not merely acknowledge the impossibility for the psychotic patient to access the depressive position. In this instance he insists that the analyst must always address a person in whom a nucleus of healthy functioning can be recognized. He underscores how psychotic patients tend to expel, through projective identification, precisely the "healthy" part of themselves, depositing it into the analyst. Should the latter unconsciously collude with this dynamic, he runs the risk of fostering a severe and potentially uncontrollable regression.

In this context, Bion recalls the contribution of Murits Katan, a Dutch analyst who had emigrated to the United States, and who was the first to describe the existence of a non-psychotic part of the personality in the schizophrenic. This insight would prove decisive, for it anticipated Bion's own formulation of the distinction between the healthy and the psychotic part of the personality: a conceptualization of fundamental importance for analytic technique as applied to psychosis.

Starting from this point, I myself will later develop some considerations on the difference between the psychotic and the healthy part of the personality: what is the true nature of the psychotic part of the personality? In what ways does it differ from the healthy part? And why does it sometimes appear so powerful as to escape any form of containment?

"The Development of Schizophrenic Thought" (1956); "Differentiation of the Psychotic from the Non-Psychotic Personalities" (1957)

In these two writings, Bion reiterates that psychosis is essentially defined by the predominance of attacks against the perception of reality. The relationship with the analyst takes on premature and precipitous features, dominated by the massive use of projective identification. To escape the risk of confusion, the patient tends to restrict the relational field to an extremely limited domain, to the point of behaving as if the analyst did not exist.

The sadistic attacks originally directed, in infantile fantasy, against the maternal breast are now displaced in the adult onto the perceptual apparatus: it is struck, fragmented, and finally expelled through projective identification. In this way, the patient destroys the very means that would have allowed him to experience reality.

At this point, the patient realizes that he has become imprisoned in the very mental condition toward which he had unconsciously gravitated. The illusion of finding in it refuge or protection now turns into an experience of captivity: he discovers that he no longer possesses that apparatus of reality-consciousness which alone could have provided him with a way out, an access to the freedom he now desires.

In other words, the psychotic mind ends up confined within the false realities it has constructed: closed and deceptive inner worlds which not only fail to sustain him, but separate him even more radically from shared reality.

The only instrument capable of orienting him toward psychic truth has dissolved. The collapse of the delusional identity leaves behind an unbearable void. The exit from psychotic withdrawal does not appear as a liberation, but as a catastrophic breakdown: the irruption of psychic reality is experienced as a trauma, an opening of the abyss of anxiety.

The parts of the perceptual apparatus, once fragmented and expelled, are fixed into external objects that continue to exist in an autonomous and uncontrollable manner. The patient perceives them as hostile, animated by a persecutory intention toward the psyche that expelled them. Thus, he feels surrounded by what Bion calls *bizarre objects*.

The bizarre object is composed of an external particle that incorporates within itself a fragment of personality. In the patient's mind, it may take on different forms: a stalker who constantly observes him, an entity that listens to and records his thoughts, a silent but relentless persecutor. This occurs because the expelled particles contain fragments of consciousness, and thus act as objects endowed with an autonomous vitality.

From this dynamic arise particularly painful hallucinatory experiences: voices that pursue the patient, intrusive tactile sensations, visual images that encircle him. Words themselves lose their symbolic nature and are treated as concrete objects—fragments of matter rather than vehicles of meaning.

The patient's inner world no longer has the dreamlike quality of the unconscious, but turns instead into a material environment populated by tangible objects, governed by physical rather than psychic laws. It is this process of materialization that makes repair so arduous, for the symbolic work of analysis collides with a universe of things rather than of thoughts.

Neurosis and Psychosis

Here Bion formulates a crucial point of distinction between neurosis and psychosis. He argues that, while the non-psychotic individual makes use of *repression*, the psychotic individual relies on *projective identification*—two mutually incompatible mechanisms.

This means that, if the psychotic needs to banish something from consciousness, he eliminates the very apparatus that would allow the psyche to carry out repression.

On this point, there is a striking convergence with Paul Federn (1952). Although starting from very different theoretical premises, Federn also observed that the psychotic patient cannot employ repression in the same way as the neurotic. For this reason, his unconscious does not operate dynamically.

In other words, whereas the neurotic can render distressing thoughts and emotions unconscious, the psychotic lacks this defensive mechanism capable of keeping overwhelming internal material at a distance—an absence that constitutes an additional complication of his mental functioning. Hence Federn's emphasis on the specificity of psychosis and the need for a radically different therapeutic approach: "in neuroses we want to lift repression, in psychoses we want to create repression" (1952, p. 136). The aim, therefore, is not to "make the unconscious conscious," but rather to "make the unconscious unconscious again" (p. 178).

If we consider what Bion would later elaborate on the role of repression within his theory of thinking, Federn's observation becomes particularly illuminating. Bion would show that repression channels sensory elements toward the alpha function, thereby rendering them thinkable and transformable into dream elements. Where this process is disrupted—as happens in psychosis through the destructive use of projective identification—the patient is unable either to dream or to think.

In this moment Bion insists forcefully on the attack the patient directs against the psychic apparatus responsible for the perception of reality. The perceptual ego is assaulted, the sense organs fragmented and expelled, orbiting around the patient like deranged satellites. The original destructiveness, born as a defense against frustration and pain, turns into a paradox: the very instrument that makes perception of reality possible is annihilated.

Psychotic and Non-Psychotic Part

A point of radical importance in these two writings is Bion's formulation of the distinction between the *psychotic and the non-psychotic part of the personality*. With this, he emphasizes that even in patients diagnosed as psychotic there always exists a healthy nucleus, one that cannot express itself because it is overwhelmed by the psychotic part. This distinction would become cardinal for clinical orientation, for it shifts the focus from the idea of a globally compromised personality to the possibility of contacting and supporting, through analysis, the healthy part that remains overshadowed.

Murits Katan (1954) was the first to speak of a non-psychotic part of the personality. Katan focused on the pre-psychotic phase of the illness, during which a part of the personality still retains the ability to manage internal conflicts and maintain contact with reality (Katan, 1954, p. 126). In this early phase, the balance between the psychotic and non-psychotic parts has not yet been fully disrupted, allowing for some degree of a reality check.

Katan further observed that psychosis may sometimes be triggered by a dream. He noted that in certain cases, dreams not only propel the dreamer into a psychotic state but may also become integrated into the delusional experience, influencing psychotic behavior.

Bion identifies the psychotic part of the personality with the destructive action of excessive projective identification, capable of dismantling and annihilating the apparatus of thought:

> the differentiation of the psychotic from the non-psychotic personalities depends on a minute splitting of all that part of the personality that is concerned with awareness of internal and external reality, and the expulsion of these fragments so that they enter into or engulf their objects.
>
> (Bion, 1957, p. 266)

The psychotic part engages in violent projections, attempting to expel psychic elements that it cannot "digest" or process, and is unable to tolerate frustration and the absence of the object. This intolerance of frustration is closely tied to excessive envy, identified as a key factor in psychotic functioning, particularly in early childhood.

For Bion, the differentiation between the psychotic and the non-psychotic parts of the personality begins in the very earliest moments of psychic life. The ongoing sadistic attacks directed against the ego and against the very matrices of thought progressively widen the distance between the two parts, until, in certain cases, it becomes irreparable. The split then turns into a radical fracture.

Excessive envy leads to a deep hatred of any relational connection. This manifests as an *attack on linking*, a destructive process that disrupts the capacity for symbolic thought and the formation of meaning. By destroying the symbolic language required to establish connections between experiences, this attack renders the psychotic mind incapable of integrating and interpreting reality.

According to Bion, it is not possible to treat a psychotic patient without analytically addressing his destructive attacks against the ego and without clarifying, again and again, the perceptual distortions produced by projective identification. The difference from the neurotic is radical: whereas the latter, through repression, maintains the possibility of "dreaming" repressed contents, the psychotic patient, by resorting to projective identification, annihilates the very organ of consciousness that would make dreaming and symbolic functioning possible.

The therapeutic obstacle therefore derives from the pervasive action of the psychotic part of the personality, which ends up determining the subject's destiny. The destructive attack fixes the patient in the schizoparanoid position, where thought processes are assaulted and deformed at their very inception. This prevents the construction of a foundation on which verbal language—and with it the entire symbolic process—could develop.

From this perspective, Bion identifies three primitive factors that contribute to destroying the possibility of a vital encounter with the object: the attack on linking, envy, and arrogance. These operate as disintegrative forces that not only obstruct conviviality with the object, but also bar access to the world of symbols and of shared emotions.

It is precisely the attack on linking that destroys the symbolic language capable of generating meaning. In this way, the possibility of establishing generative pairings, of creating connections that transform sensory experience into living thought, is nullified. Intolerance of frustration, which Bion associates with excessive envy present from the earliest phases of life, gives rise to a radical hatred toward every form of connection: between mother and child, between analyst and patient, between different parts of the self. This is the attack on linking that undermines the very possibility of thinking.

Bion's technique consists in interpreting directly to the patient his destructive operations, describing the ways in which he uses his psychic and bodily organs, continually fragmented, expelled, and transformed into bizarre objects.

When the patient attempts to restore a minimum of ego cohesion and to reclaim these fragments, he must resort to a kind of "reverse" projective identification, retracing the same path through which the parts were expelled. Yet he cannot truly reintegrate these fragments: he can only glue them together in a mechanical way. If, moreover, he perceives the analyst as one who seeks to reintegrate them from the outside, he experiences such intervention as an act of violence and intrusion.

Interpreting from Above

As I have already mentioned, Bion's interpretations may at times appear as if they were "falling from above." He himself, reflecting retrospectively on his work, acknowledged that on some occasions his interpretations arose from theory even before clinical material.

At one point he explicitly states:

> I shall now attempt a description of an actual session; it is a clinical experience based on these theories rather than the description of an experience on which the theories are based, but I hope I shall be able to indicate the material from previous sessions which led me to interpret as I did.
>
> (Bion, 1957, p. 270)

It is precisely from this statement that Bion would later develop his celebrated technical recommendation to approach the patient "without memory and without desire." With this formula he sought to free the analyst both from the weight of theory and from the burden of personal expectations: memory understood as a set of already acquired schemas, and desire as the tendency to orient the encounter toward a predetermined outcome.

The analyst, Bion would later affirm, must be disposed to receive what occurs in the session without anticipating it and without forcing it into already familiar categories.

Only in this way does it become possible to truly receive the psychotic patient, who cannot be understood through a pre-established knowledge—one derived from our experience with neurotic patients—but only by attempting to grasp the patient's communication, which can make use solely of a mode situated outside dynamic unconscious processes, repression, and symbolization.

I will now present the sequence of a session in which it seems to me that Bion interprets from above.

Bion speaks of a psychotic patient, enigmatic and almost always silent, who had been in analysis for six years. The patient had repeatedly said that for him analysis was a torture of memories, and that therefore, when he suffered, he sought anesthesia, as if only the abolition of memory could free him from pain.

During the session, after declaring that his head was splitting, he suddenly exclaimed: "It must be the dark glasses!"

Bion then recalled that about nine months earlier he had come into session wearing dark glasses, and that this image had been imprinted in the patient's mind as a fragment expelled from the ego, transformed into a bizarre object.

The phrase about the headache and the glasses thus appeared to him as the attempt of the psychotic part of the personality to construct an ideogram: a raw thought, expressed not in words but through a visual sign of a sensory nature.

Bion associates the glass of the spectacles with the feeding bottle, and the two lenses with the maternal breast. Being made of glass, the lenses would represent the possibility of being pierced by the patient's aggressiveness when he attacks the breast. Their dark color, instead, would allude to threat and persecutory rage.

The glasses are dark because darkness, in unconscious fantasy, is required in order to spy on the parents during the sexual act. The patient also refers to having swallowed the feeding bottle together with the milk, with the consequence that even good objects become black, transformed into ominous and persecutory objects.

The dark glasses thus come to assume the meaning of a persecutory conscience that punishes the patient: on the one hand because he uses them to abolish pain, on the other because he employs them, in fantasy, to spy on the analyst and on the parents in their sexual union.

Starting from these associations, Bion interprets that the patient had taken back sight inside himself, but that this now split his head open, since it was perceived as profoundly bad, for the maltreatment it had inflicted on him. To this interpretation the patient replied only: "Nothing," arching his back. Bion responded: "Nothing seems like your back," and the patient added: "Moral constraints."

The dialogue highlights the difficulty of translating inner experience into words, an experience that remains conveyed through bodily and postural forms. In this sequence Bion considers that, in the psychotic condition, the ego's reparative process implies a return to primitive preverbal modes, damaged by mutilations and projective identifications. The dark glasses thus represent an agglomerate of bizarre objects: a composite of expelled fragments sufficiently organized to function as a means of communication.

As can be observed, Bion's clinical work does not rest on the patient's free associations—which, in the case of the psychotic, are virtually absent—but on attention to the deep mechanisms he identifies as nuclei of pathological transformation: hatred of the breast, excessive use of projective identification, the formation of bizarre objects, envy of the parental coitus, guilt, and the action of a persecutory Superego.

In Bion's evaluation, the outcome of the session—which I have here summarized in concise form—was positive. The patient showed a tangible improvement, expressed both in the more frequent use of verbal thought and in a more benevolent attitude toward the analyst. Bion attributes this change to the fact that the patient was able to reduce his destructive attacks against the ego and to recover, at least in part, the possibility of employing repression in place of projective identification.

"On Hallucination" (1958)

In this paper Bion describes a psychotic patient who had been in analysis for several years, punctual and regular in his attendance. As he lies down on the couch, Bion notices that the patient reproduces, with striking synchrony, each of his gestures, as if analyst and patient were cogs within the same clockwork mechanism. Once prone, the patient fixes his gaze insistently on a corner of the room.

Bion hypothesizes that, upon entering, the patient had captured him with his eyes—used as an organ of suction—and then expelled him into that corner, where he now kept him under a fixed stare. From this perspective the sensory organ is not merely an instrument of reception but also a vehicle of projection.

The expulsive process, Bion observes, may manifest in different modalities: through sight in visual hallucinations, through the ears in auditory ones, through the skin in tactile phenomena. Here the hallucinatory state appears as the consequence of the hatred expressed by the patient at the end of the previous session. The hallucination would therefore represent the attempt to evacuate, via the eyes, that hostile nucleus lodged in the mind that had become intolerable.

In this case, Bion interprets the split, the hallucination, and the use of sight as an expulsive organ as having a meaning distinct from the patient's usual acts of violent, parceled fragmentation. He believes, in fact, that the patient is coming into contact with an internal bad object and is now attempting to eject it. The convulsive movements that follow the interpretation seem to indicate that the analyst's words were experienced as a persecutory intrusion: the patient perceives the analyst as the one who violently returns to him the very aggressive emotions he had projected.

If this session, by the patient's own acknowledgment, can be regarded as positive, the next one shows no favorable development. The patient becomes incoherent and dissociated: he reports having ordered a coffee shortly before arriving, but having felt that the barista bore him a grudge, perhaps because of his voice; he also recounts that, while passing through the gate, the bars seemed to dilate, only to find on his way back that everything remained unchanged.

Faced with these alarming statements, Bion offers no immediate comment. The patient continues to speak, but with sentences that seem meaningless. The analyst points out the vacuity of his discourse; the patient replies that he had "put his gramophone in that place." Bion then thinks that with this image the patient was communicating his perception of the analyst's interpretations as records he knows by heart, and that for this reason he had expelled them—"defecating them."

At a certain point the atmosphere of the session changes: the patient feels anguished, experiences a sense of emptiness, and becomes persecutory.

He says, "I have to use my ears. I seem to hear things all wrong." This time the analyst's words do not slide off him but penetrate his ears in a way that for him is "all wrong," that is, with a cruel and destructive meaning.

Bion hypothesizes that his interpretations were seized and assimilated by the ears and then expelled through the eyes, and he says to him: "You are feeling that your ears are chewing up and destroying all that I say to you. You are so anxious to get rid of it that you at once expel the pieces out of your eyes."

The patient continues: "All sounds turn into things I see around me." Bion interprets that he is again turning interpretations into sounds and then evacuating them through his eyes, so that he now perceives them as objects surrounding him.

The clinical sequence clearly highlights the way in which Bion works with the psychotic patient in the analytic setting. He maintains that the psychotic part is constantly active during the session and can always become the object of interpretation. Yet the impact of destructive attacks is such that the patient is left bereft of verbal thought, with a fragmented ego. What survives are only shards, splinters of thought: the analyst thus finds himself before the wreckage of a ship destroyed at sea, which he must attempt to reassemble.

The analyst's task consists in recognizing these fragments and trying to stitch them together into a configuration that might restore a semblance of ego. But the work is arduous, for the patient lacks any integrative function: the objects, even when they appear to cluster, never truly cohere, and often develop a centrifugal force that pulls them further apart.

Analysis therefore unfolds within a continuous projective exchange between patient and analyst, in which fragments of the ego are deposited, evacuated, and at times momentarily repositioned.

A crucial question then arises: to whom is the analyst addressing himself? To which part of the patient does he speak?

Bion richly describes the functioning of the psychotic part—its hatred of reality, the fragmentation of ego and objects, the inner persecution—but devotes far less space to the role of the non-psychotic part, which does exist, albeit in a diminished and minority form.

The resulting style of analytic work resembles that of one attempting to gather together the shards of a broken vase, without, however, possessing any adhesive to fix them. The aim remains that of helping the patient to integrate scattered fragments; yet the fragments, when brought close to one another, tend to repel, as though an inner force were preventing any stable recomposition.

As I will try to outline later on, it will take many years of clinical work and thoughtful reflection—also by other pioneers in the field of psychoanalysis—to envisage a viable path toward integration. Such a process must begin not only with a clear understanding of the origins and psychopathology of psychotic illness, but also with the formation of an alliance between the patient's healthy part and the analyst's sustained and vigilant awareness on the psychotic part's power to invade and dominate the rest of the personality.

Chapter 3

Bion's Second Phase

"Attacks on Linking" (1959)

Up to this point, I have outlined the theoretical framework that characterized the first phase of Bion's work on psychosis: a perspective centered on destructiveness, on hatred toward reality, and on the difficulty of any reparative attempt.

In "Attacks on Linking" (1959), he still insists above all on the psychotic patient's hatred of reality and of every form of link, underlining the destructive force that aims to break any connection.

To demonstrate his thesis, Bion recounts the case of one of his patients. After much of the session had passed in silence, the patient suddenly announced that a piece of iron had fallen to the floor. Immediately afterward, he began to make convulsive movements, as if assaulted from within. Bion interpreted that the patient could not establish contact with him because he was terrified by what he felt inside himself. The patient confirmed this: he had the sensation of being murdered.

Bion added that the envy directed toward himself and toward the analyst—for the possibility of working together—was so intense that it drove him to introject them as a piece of dead iron and a dead floor, joined not to give him life, but to kill him.

At that point the patient, overwhelmed by anguish, said that he could not continue. Bion told him that he was unable to go on because he already felt dead, or else alive but so envious that he had to interrupt any possibility of a good analysis.

A Change of Perspective

After having insisted almost to the point of excess on the indispensable importance of projective identification in the psychotic process, Bion (p. 312) then introduces an unexpected reversal of perspective.

Bion opens himself to a series of insights that mark a radical change—a true revolution capable of profoundly altering the very way in which analytic

DOI: 10.4324/9781003765363-4

technique and the analyst's clinical function are conceived. This concerns his new understanding of projective identification: no longer only as an evacuative and destructive mechanism, but also as a channel of primitive communication between patient and analyst.

Melanie Klein had not foreseen this possibility and, as some of her collaborators recalled, even regretted not having grasped it. With Bion, the analyst's task is no longer limited to interpreting in order to make the patient aware of his functioning and aggressive aspects; he must also receive the communication and contain the anxiety transmitted by the patient, take it into himself, and return it in a transformed form, capable of being assimilated.

In Bion's new perspective, projective identification is not only a means of expelling what is intolerable, but also becomes a vehicle of communication. The analyst—like a sufficiently good mother—must internalize the patient's projection, give it a shape, a name, and return it in a transformed manner so that it may be assimilated.

To carry out this task, both the mother and the analyst are called to a specific kind of work: they must identify with the child or the patient, placing themselves in their position in order to understand them—an operation that a psychotic patient, enclosed within their own sensory world, will never be able to perform.

This redefinition of the concept of projective identification marks a decisive turning point: it offers analytic technique a different mode of working, more relational and empathic, and profoundly alters the very meaning of interpretation and of the analytic role.

The analyst thus becomes a transformational object (Bollas, 1987), and no longer merely the one who interprets and makes the unconscious manifest.

Bion recounts a session in which he had repeatedly interpreted to another patient the attempt to rid himself of intolerable annihilation anxieties by projecting them onto the analyst. Only later did he realize that the patient was not using projective identification as an attack, but rather as an act of trust: he was handing over his anxieties in the hope that they might be transformed and returned in a more tolerable form.

Since Bion had been unable to contain and share the anxiety, the patient's effort to re-project it into the analyst became increasingly desperate: the more violent his projections, the more terrifying the image of the analyst became in his eyes.

The words Bion employs to describe this experience are particularly moving:

> Associations from a period in the analysis earlier than that from which these illustrations have been drawn showed an increasing intensity of emotions in the patient. This originated in what he felt was my refusal to accept parts of his personality. Consequently, he strove to force them into me with increased desperation and violence. His behaviour, isolated from the context of the analysis, might have appeared to be an expression of primary aggression. The more violent his phantasies of projective

> identification, the more frightened he became of me. There were sessions in which such behaviour expressed unprovoked aggression, but I quote this series because it shows the patient in a different light, his violence a reaction to what he felt was my hostile defensiveness. The analytic situation built up in my mind a sense of witnessing an extremely early scene. I felt that the patient had experienced in infancy a mother who dutifully responded to the infant's emotional displays. The dutiful response had in it an element of impatient "I don't know what's the matter with the child." My deduction was that in order to understand what the child wanted the mother should have treated the infant's cry as more than a demand for her presence. From the infant's point of view she should have taken into her, and thus experienced, the fear that the child was dying. It was this fear that the child could not contain. He strove to split it off together with the part of the personality in which it lay and project it into the mother. An understanding mother is able to experience the feeling of dread, that this baby was striving to deal with by projective identification, and yet retain a balanced outlook. This patient had had to deal with a mother who could not tolerate experiencing such feelings and reacted either by shutting them out, or alternatively by becoming a prey to the anxiety which resulted from introjection of the infant's feelings. The latter reaction, I think, must have been rare: denial was dominant.
>
> (p. 312)

It is striking that such statements appear precisely in a text devoted to the attack on linking. Up to that point, in fact, Bion had understood projective identification exclusively as a destructive movement, an expression of the psychotic part of the personality.

Suddenly, however, he introduces a conceptual shift: he theorizes the existence of a "normal," or better, communicative form of projective identification which, like introjection, becomes a primary condition for mental growth and psychic development.

From this perspective, the patient does not expel fragments of his own personality with the aim of appropriating those of the object—as in Klein's example of Fabien—but rather transmits emotions that ask to be understood, worked through, and then returned.

Here lies the radical difference between the two modalities of projective identification: one destructive and colonizing, the other communicative and transformative.

The Maternal Container

It is precisely this intuition of Bion—that projective identification can function as a communicative bridge—that forms the foundation of his elaboration on the *container–contained* relationship, a theoretical cornerstone for understanding emotional growth and the process of psychic development.

From this angle, Bion observes, even aggressiveness assumes a new meaning. In the session, the patient may feel gratitude for the analytic opportunity offered to him, and at the same time hate the analyst, perceived as the one who will reject the only language at his disposal. Destructive attacks, rooted in infantile deprivations, thus come to appear as though they originated more from the analyst than from the patient himself.

For the first time, throughout his work with psychotic patients, Bion moves beyond the idea of innate destructiveness, formulating the hypothesis of an emotionally traumatic condition.

If projective identification represents, for the child, the means by which he comes to understand the nature of his emotions—by seeing how they are received and worked through by the mother—then a mother unable to receive such communication creates instead the very conditions for the destruction of emotional life.

Although he had this fertile intuition—which he would later develop into the concept of maternal and analytic *reverie*—Bion, when dealing with psychotic patients, did not at first seem to grasp its full innovative significance.

In fact, despite this fertile intuition, Bion remains suspended: he does not fully recognize the innovative scope of his hypothesis, nor does he ascribe to this primary experience of relational trauma the principal matrix of psychosis. Rather, he continues to locate the original factors in the child's aggressiveness and envy. Even while taking maternal unresponsiveness into account, he insists upon the infant's predisposition to hatred, aggressiveness, and envy, as if these remained the irreducible nuclei of the disorder.

In certain cases, a congenital factor may prevail; in others, however, the decisive weight falls upon the mother's insufficient receptivity. When the mother proves incapable of receiving and containing the child's projections, or when the child's hatred and envy become excessive, the consequence is the destruction of the primary bond between infant and breast.

The failure of this original encounter fosters the establishment, within the patient's inner world, of a relentless, persecutory Superego that attacks or annihilates the Ego. If the child identifies with such an object, it becomes the "bad self," a nucleus that triumphs by destroying the relationship with the object and undermining the capacity to learn from experience.

The internal object, born as a refusing breast incapable of receiving the child's emotions, is then configured as an enemy of all linking: it obstructs, poisons, and dissolves them. It is therefore not surprising that the relationships which survive such attacks retain a perverse, cruel, and sterile imprint.

Bion (1967) observes that in psychotic patients the function that should nourish curiosity has been not merely inhibited, but almost extinguished, to the point of making the very emergence of a question impossible. The incapacity to observe and to turn one's gaze upon oneself finds its most radical expression in delusion, which appears as a concrete event, not translatable into symbolic terms, not representable nor thinkable. It is, as Bion will write, an operation of the opposite sign to the creative one: a veritable experience of –K.

In my view, one of the most significant nodes in Bion's thought (1967) is his observation that the psychotic suffers from a deficit of curiosity, a function which, if only it could be reactivated, would open the way to the therapeutic process. This is not a secondary detail: curiosity represents, in fact, the very possibility of asking questions, of accessing the causal nexus that makes experience thinkable.

And it is precisely here, according to Bion, that the limit is encountered: "Another feature obtrudes if the course of the analysis is favourable; problems which in sophisticated language are posed by the question 'Why?' cannot be formulated" (p. 314).

In other words, the psychotic is trapped in a condition that prevents him not only from learning, but even from questioning.

This point leads us to consider the nature of traumatic experiences, which share with psychotic experiences the same impossibility of becoming thought. Because of the excess of anxiety, they cannot enter the unconscious, are not transformed, and consequently cannot be repressed or forgotten. Even when the psychotic crisis abates, what remains is an unprocessed nucleus, encapsulated within the psyche, ready to generate instability and possible relapses. Hence the observation of the old psychiatrists that the recoveries of psychotic states were always "defective": an improvement that does not fully integrate the personality, but leaves parts of the experience untransformed and unresolved.

At the heart of the problem lies, once again, the primary communication between mother and infant. It is in this original exchange that the trauma is located.

Bion writes:

> Projective identification makes it possible for him to investigate his own feelings in a personality powerful enough to contain them. Denial of the use of this mechanism, either by the refusal of the mother to serve as a repository for the infant's feelings, or by the hatred and envy of the patient who cannot allow the mother to exercise this function, leads to a destruction of the link between infant and breast and consequently to a severe disorder of the impulse to be curious on which all learning depends. The way is therefore prepared for a severe arrest of development.
>
> (p. 312)

This passage is decisive: the mother's failure to contain does not merely undermine the child's capacity to tolerate his own emotions, but directly impedes the development of curiosity—that vital impulse which makes it possible to learn from experience.

From this original arrest a vicious circle emerges: instead of opening toward thought, emotion calls forth hatred, and from hatred toward emotional life the step to hatred toward life itself becomes inexorably brief.

It is natural to ask why Bion, after grasping the vital importance of communicative projective identification and the receptive function of the maternal mind, nonetheless continued to uphold the constitutional and destructive hypothesis of the illness. Is it not plausible that the bond of fidelity which tied him to Melanie Klein restrained him?

It is legitimate to think that it was precisely the fear of an irreparable conflict with her that led him not to carry through the consequences of his most radical intuitions.

Looking more closely, the crucial point is clear: when the mother fails in her receptive function, the embryonic consciousness of the infant is forced to take upon itself an impossible task—that which the mother has not been able to accomplish.

Analysis shows us that the psychotic patient, at bottom, finds himself reliving this same legacy: he carries within, like a mark, the incapacity of the internal object to receive and give meaning to his emotions.

With the passage of time, it has become possible to understand more clearly the reasons why Bion was unable to resolve the dilemma as to whether the origin of psychosis should be attributed to the predominance of the destructive drive or to a deficit in maternal reverie.

My hypothesis is that the absence of maternal reverie alone is not sufficient to generate infantile sensory withdrawal, which, as I shall explain later, constitutes a psychopathological structure created by the child himself as an alternative to the failed communication with the mother, and which nourishes the psychotic part of the personality.

At the time Bion was writing, the concept of psychopathological structures had not yet been formulated.

Chapter 4

A Theory of Thinking

After the works previously discussed, Bion would provide only rare accounts of his clinical engagement with psychotic patients. Gradually, his focus shifted toward the theory of thinking—a theme that would accompany him for many years and, in broadening his perspective, lead him to profound and radical insights into the distinction between intuitive thought and psychotic thought.

The beginning of this trajectory is marked by "The Psycho-Analytic Study of Thinking" (1962b) presented at the Edinburgh Congress in 1961, published the following year in the *International Journal of Psychoanalysis*, and later revisited in *Second Thoughts*.

Bion writes:

> Thoughts may be classified, according to the nature of their developmental history, as pre-conceptions, conceptions or thoughts, and finally concepts; concepts are named and therefore fixed conceptions or thoughts. The conception is initiated by the conjunction of a pre-conception with a realization.

The infant, for example, possesses the pre-conception of the existence of a breast.

> When the pre-conception is brought into contact with a realization that approximates to it, the mental outcome is a conception. Put in another way, the pre-conception (the inborn expectation of a breast, the a priori knowledge of a breast, the "empty thought") when the infant is brought in contact with the breast itself, mates with awareness of the realization and is synchronous with the development of a conception. This model will serve for the theory that every junction of a pre-conception with its realization produces a conception.
>
> (Bion, 1962b, p. 305)

It follows that conceptions are necessarily linked to the experience of satisfaction.

DOI: 10.4324/9781003765363-5

The meaning of the term "thinking," however, arises from the conjunction of an idea with frustration. If the infant's expectation of a breast does not find realization, two possibilities emerge: either the child succeeds in tolerating frustration and in transforming it, or he will attempt to flee from a condition experienced as intolerable.

The capacity to endure absence allows the psyche to think, in order to fill the space left vacant by the missing object. When this capacity fails, the outcome is the creation of a bad object, destined solely for expulsion. In this way, the development of the apparatus for thinking is arrested, leaving evacuation as the only possible outcome.

This second apparatus functions according to the principle that there is no difference between evacuating a bad breast and drawing comfort from a good breast.

The inability to tolerate frustration generates a defensive omnipotence that seeks to eliminate all experiences arising from the encounter between a pre-conception and a negative realization. In extreme cases, in order to avoid such an encounter, the subject may go so far as to annihilate the very existence of space and time.

Alpha-Function

At this point (p. 308), Bion introduces the concept of the *alpha-function*, the function entrusted with transforming sensory impressions into alpha-elements, indispensable for the production of dream thoughts. If, within the mother–infant relationship, normal projective identification is lacking, the alpha-function fails to develop, and with it also the possibility of distinguishing between conscious and unconscious contents.

The infant, in fact, is incapable of autonomously transforming sensory impressions: he can only evacuate them into the mother, entrusting her with the operations necessary to render them usable as alpha-elements. The transformative capacity of sensory data depends upon maternal *reverie*, which—if absent—prevents the passage from the sensory to the psychic, and deprives the child's projective identifications of meaning.

At this stage, it is particularly useful to turn to *Cogitations* (1992), a collection of notes that Bion left behind during the course of his work.

One of the central themes in *Cogitations* concerns the work of the *alpha dream*. With this expression Bion designates the set of operations through which the subject transforms sensory impressions into elements of thought.

This process unfolds in two stages: the first, of an analytic nature, consists in breaking down sensory data into simple, incoherent ideograms; the second, of a synthetic nature, confers structure upon this fragmentary material, thereby rendering the sensory impression both memorable and communicable.

These two phases correspond, in psychoanalytic terms, to the transition from the schizoparanoid position to the depressive position: from the disintegration of sensory data to their integration—a process that enables the formation of memory and of the unconscious.

In the section "Tropisms" of *Cogitations*, Bion states that the development of personality depends upon the existence of an object analogous to the breast, into which tropisms (that is, projective identifications) can be deposited. Where such an object is absent, the destiny of the personality is marked by catastrophe: the loss of contact with reality, manifesting as apathy or mania.

From this premise, Bion highlights how the failure to develop certain fundamental functions of affective symbolization derives from a defect in the container—that primary object originally destined to receive the infant's projections, embodied in a mother deprived of *reverie* and, consequently, of alpha-function.

For Bion, to memorize a sensory impression means first and foremost to render it unconscious, thereby creating a distinction between conscious and unconscious. He distinguishes *alpha-dream-work* from the Freudian concept of dream-work, understood as the process that, by overcoming repression, allows repressed contents to become manifest.

Bion does not attribute this function to repression: in his view, repression is not the matrix of the dream, but rather a necessary step that allows the work of the alpha dream to operate, and thus permits thought to emerge.

Earlier, Bion had approached this idea, observing how the psychotic, unlike the "normal" individual, is unable to make use of repression and therefore lacks a true unconscious life and operates primarily through projective mechanisms. From this it follows that the psychotic cannot think: he lacks, in fact, an apparatus capable of transforming sensory experiences into thoughts, which is why his mind remains confined to *beta-elements.*

If the transition from beta to alpha occurs within the dream, this transformation is barred to the psychotic, who remains bound to a sensory use of the mind: he remains a constructor of images and narratives, not one who dreams but one who builds concrete, non-symbolic worlds. In his case, beta-elements are produced by the psychotic part of the personality and, as such, are not transformable, since they derive from the inversion of the alpha-function.

In this condition, frustration becomes increasingly intolerable for the psychotic, precisely because he progressively distances himself from the only instrument that might relieve it: the capacity to think. Indeed, the psychotic cannot escape from the prison he has constructed for himself, for he has destroyed the very means that might liberate him.

Chapter 5

Hallucination

In "On Hallucination" (1958), Bion observes that the sense organs—normally devoted to perception, recognition, and the identification of objects—become instruments of evacuation for products and fragments generated by the process of hallucinatory transformation. Evacuation through the sensory organs may manifest in visual, auditory, olfactory, or tactile hallucinations, which are not always clinically evident.

In the hallucinatory transformation, the patient tends to believe that his own "creations" derive from the attainment of a privileged condition, superior to any other psychic experience.

This state is felt as extraordinarily blissful and precious, to the extent that he fears the analyst might deprive him of it. Analysis is therefore perceived as a threat: an attempt to rob him of that state of supremacy, of that exceptional capacity which he experiences as the most exhilarating core of his psychic life.

Bion emphasizes that, in constructing the hallucinatory world, the patient abolishes every form of dependence upon the analyst and upon the external world, since he perceives himself as capable of creating anything autonomously. In this way, frustration is eliminated and envy nullified: his greed is always satisfied, for every need can be gratified through the hallucinatory method.

In *Transformations* (1965), he stresses once again that hallucination, in this perspective, no longer moves within the three-dimensional space of rigid-motion transformations nor within the multi-dimensional space of projective transformations: it is situated in an infinite space, without coordinates or dimensions, because it originates from the destruction of the container. It is a dimension in which space and time are annihilated by the psychotic part of the personality.

As a consequence, psychic contents, things-in-themselves, and beta-elements remain free, raw, and untransformed.

To illustrate this process, Bion resorts to abstract signs such as the point (.) and the line (–). These symbols may represent space and time, fundamental categories for situating objects and object relations. For instance, (.) and (–) may indicate the position that an object, perceived by the non-psychotic part of the personality, occupies in space and time when it is absent.

DOI: 10.4324/9781003765363-6

The psychotic part, incapable of tolerating absence, through the hallucinatory transformation inverts the temporal sequence "not now" and the spatial sequence "not here" into their opposite: "here-now-it is." In this way, a space populated by non-existent objects is created—sometimes through actual hallucinations, at other times through equivalent phenomena, evanescent and invisible, but no less binding upon the subject's experience.

This insight of Bion's is of considerable significance and explains why the psychotic is unable to use the mind in an intuitive and creative mode.

For Bion, the possibility of using the mind to develop thought presupposes the absence of sensory perceptions. According to Bion, thought arises only where psychic space is not saturated by sensory perceptions: the inner void, far from being a threat, becomes the very condition of possibility for symbolic activity. In psychosis, by contrast, perceptions transformed into hallucinations occupy the entire mental space, obstructing any process of creative elaboration.

Although hallucinations may involve any of the senses (sight, hearing, touch, smell, and taste), the most studied and commonly occurring are auditory. In psychotic patients hallucinations tend to be an expression of a delusional system.

Important in the study of hallucinations is the judgment of reality: How does the patient assign reality to stimuli that, beyond all reasonable doubt, originate in his mind?

Hallucination is the result of a mental operation that destroys alpha-elements (symbols), reducing them to fragments that can only be evacuated but not thought.

This evacuation occurs through sense organs whose functioning is reversed so that digested beta-elements are expelled into the external world together with traces of the Ego and Superego, thus giving rise to bizarre objects.

Sometimes, transformations in hallucinosis do not involve the perception of non-existent objects but the perception of non-existent relations.

As I will discuss in detail later, my clinical hypothesis is that hallucinatory phenomena are the result of a distorted use of the mind practiced over a long period by the psychotic outside his awareness: instead of being a tool for relating with others—that is, an organ of knowledge—the mind is employed to create a sensory world dominated by a special, regressive type of pleasure.

And this is how the primitive infantile withdrawal into the world of sensory fantasies is created (De Masi, 2020).

Since hallucinations have a "sensory" and concrete quality, they can easily deceive the patient as they are similar to perceptions that, under normal conditions, describe the surrounding world. Put differently, visual hallucinations arise from seeing with the mind's "eyes" and auditory hallucinations from hearing with the mind's "ears."

The hallucinatory symptom originates in such clear and indisputable sensory perceptions that any recourse to normal experiences that confirm reality would be in vain. In other words, hallucinations are "prepared" by the psychotic part that seduces and dominates the patient.

The mind is not employed to think but to see and hear, that is, it functions according to sensory images, to perceptions–thoughts.

For this reason, hallucinations and delusions cannot be investigated as if they were dreams, fantasies, or thoughts, using tools appropriate in the neuroses, that is, interpretations. It is, however, possible to investigate the ways in which the psychotic patient creates these.

Usually the psychotic hallucinatory experience is positive and seducing in the beginning, with gentle, charming voices, but it then changes, with critical, contemptuous, and terrifying voices coming onto the scene, and the state of grandiosity gradually turns into a condition of persecution.

Chapter 6

Further Developments

After the publication of *Second Thoughts*, Bion devoted himself with rigor to logical and epistemological reflection, aiming to confer a more rigorous status upon psychoanalysis. His references to psychosis, although moving away from direct clinical experience, were reinterpreted in the light of his theoretical elaborations, thereby acquiring a deeper and more expressive significance.

Learning from Experience (1962a)

In this work Bion revisits the central hypothesis of the transformation of sensory impressions into thought. It is the alpha-function that operates this transformation: through the proliferation of alpha-elements, it constructs the contact-barrier, which serves simultaneously as a surface of separation and as a point of communication between conscious and unconscious.

This barrier guarantees the rhythm between sleep and wakefulness, the possibility of self-awareness, and the experience of shared reality.

When the alpha-function fails, beta-elements accumulate and give rise to the beta-screen: an "aggregate of things-in-themselves" which, being untransformable, produces disarticulation of language, confusional states, and hallucinatory phenomena.

Onto this screen malformed alpha-elements may at times become grafted, transforming into "bizarre objects" that carry traces of the Ego and the Superego. Although Bion does not state it explicitly, it is evident that the beta-screen and the proliferation of its elements characterize the mind of the psychotic, who is unable to transform them and is therefore exposed to catastrophic outcomes.

It is based on these reflections that Bion reconsiders the problem of the original disposition to psychosis. He maintains that, if a child possesses a sufficient capacity to tolerate frustration, he or she can survive even the devastating experience of a mother incapable of *reverie.*

Conversely, if tolerance of frustration is gravely compromised, the absence of maternal *reverie* produces a psychic collapse.

Here an unresolved question arises: if, as Bion himself insists, maternal *reverie* and the alpha-function are indispensable conditions for normal

DOI: 10.4324/9781003765363-7

development, how can he hypothesize that a child might dispense with them, relying on a sort of innate resilience? On this point, various authors have taken position.

Meltzer, for example, insisted that maternal *reverie* is not an accessory but a structuring function: without it, thought cannot be born.

Green, with his theory of the "dead mother," emphasized that the absence of maternal *reverie* always produces a traumatic experience, for which no internal reserve of frustration tolerance can truly compensate.

Winnicott too, though in a different register, stressed that without a sufficiently containing environment the child develops no genuine continuity of existence: intrapsychic strength alone is not enough if the external function of holding is lacking.

In this sense, Bion's indeterminacy seems to mark the sign of an unresolved tension. On the one hand, he seeks to formulate universal principles, such as the indispensability of *reverie*; on the other, he does not appear fully convinced that communicative projective identification always requires a response, and that this is the only viable path for development.

It is as if Bion were unable to relinquish the first hypothesis advanced in his theory of thinking, in which the capacity to tolerate frustration—a near-innate function—enables the psyche to formulate thoughts that fill the space left vacant by the absent object. His second hypothesis, by contrast, highlights the role of the maternal mind in enabling the infant to formulate thoughts by acquiring the alpha-function.

Hanna Segal (1957), moreover, had already stressed that the capacity to symbolize derives from the ability to tolerate absence—that is, from the ability to internally sustain the presence of the loved object when it is absent.

It must be emphasized that for this process to become structured, multiple experiences of felicitous encounters between the mother's mind and that of the child are necessary.

When communication—first sensory and then emotional—proves chronically deficient, the child is unable to sustain a living psychic relational life and he instead must resort to compensatory and defensive sensory experiences such as physical excitement, bodily stereotypies, compulsive masturbation, and withdrawal into sensory fantasies—all defensive modalities aimed at escaping collapse.

It seems to me that, in this case, Bion remains within a purely theoretical view of the problem concerning the dynamic between nature and culture—that is, the extent to which environmental experience, or culture, can integrate and modify the original disposition.

If we move beyond the purely theoretical domain, clinical experience shows us how essential it is to consider the relational vertex in the development of every patient. It is in fact impossible to assume the total absence of an empathic maternal response. We usually encounter partial responses, accompanied—certainly—by absences or distortions. Yet, in every case, something positive has passed between the mother's mind and that of the infant, allowing at least for survival.

And if it was not the mother who provided the child with experiences useful for development, we sometimes find that another person, in part, replaced the parental presence. We cannot forget that, in every patient we meet—even the most severely disturbed—there always exists a healthy part of the personality, and this could not have developed out of nothing.

Transformations (1965)

Here Bion returns to the theme of psychosis, shifting attention to the nature of psychic transformations.

He distinguishes two fundamental modalities: "rigid-motion" transformations and "projective" transformations, differentiated by the degree of deformation the original figure undergoes and by the possibility of recognizing its invariants. The former imply only a minimal displacement, so that the figure remains easily identifiable; the latter, by contrast, involve radical deformations, in which only the most essential properties remain stable.

Rigid-motion transformations are characteristic of neurotic processes and of transference. The analysand, in fact, reconstructs the analytic relationship by tracing it back to past experiences deposited in memory as alpha-elements.

For Bion, such transformations take place within a "Euclidean," three-dimensional mental space, regulated by Oedipal coordinates: it is indeed the Oedipal experience that renders possible the symbolization of reality and the differentiation between subject and object.

Projective transformations, on the other hand, unfold within a radically different field. They do not employ the analyst as a symbolic support for feelings and past representations; rather, they correspond to the expulsion of beta-elements through projective identification. The space in which they are produced no longer maintains geometrical coherence. They correspond, rather, to the operations of projective identification and to the evacuation of beta-elements.

This type of transformation occurs within a profoundly distorted psychic field, not only in spatial terms but also in temporal ones: events distant in time may be experienced as current, and space itself loses its Euclidean consistency. It is precisely in this disarray that one perceives the psychotic matrix of projective transformations, where the mind is invaded by expelled and untransformed contents.

Here the psychotic mind reveals its incapacity for symbolic transformation, operating instead through expulsions and distortions that generate confusion and a loss of continuity. We can observe that while in Klein projection still preserves a link with the object, in Bion the focus shifts to the catastrophic effect of the massive expulsion of beta-elements, which cannot be transformed.

For Bion, hallucination represents the most extreme point of psychic deformation. It no longer retains the three-dimensional space of rigid-motion transformations, nor the multi-dimensional field of projective transformations: it moves instead within an unlimited, coordinate-free space, the product of the destruction of the container. In this absolute dimension, both space and time are annihilated.

Unlike the neurotic personality, which accepts a certain delimitation of mental space, the psychotic personality tolerates no constraint: it experiences every limit as an unbearable prison and resorts to hallucination as a means of escaping such a condition.

In the neurotic personality, the alpha-function ensures the transformation of psychic reality into a three-dimensional space, a container that gathers together elements already thought and others yet to be thought, maintaining them in reciprocal relation. In this case, the alpha-function operates like a silent weaver: it transforms psychic reality into a structured mental space.

The condition of the psychotic personality is entirely different: according to Bion, there exists no container capable of mapping the mental state and conferring psychic consistency to experience. The elements which, in the healthy part, remain bound in a stable conjunction undergo instead a kind of "explosive projection": they are dispersed, fragmented, reduced to particles without any possibility of cohesion.

The perception of space that results is that of an immensity without representation, not even comparable to astronomical space, since any symbolic point of reference is lacking.

The intolerance of frustration and the omnipotence of the psychotic, in pursuit of absolute freedom, drive toward transformations that dissolve limits: space becomes unlimited, but such boundlessness inevitably culminates in an equally boundless panic.

What to an external observer might appear as thought, visual image, or verbalization is in reality nothing more than the residue of language and of emotional experiences already dispersed within a spaceless and timeless dimension.

The loss of the container generates a space, devoid of representational possibility.

From this perspective, hallucination is not merely a flight from containment nor simply an evacuation of beta-elements: it is the extreme outcome of a search for absolute freedom, a freedom which, instead of liberating, destroys the very psychic space itself.

The psychotic, in the illusion of escaping the prison of limitation, exposes himself to an unbounded immensity that can neither be inhabited nor represented. In this immensity, what remains of the mind is no longer thought but scattered fragments: residues of language, shards of emotion, isolated images that do not cohere into experience.

A notion akin to the boundless space generated by hallucinatory transformation is the one formulated by Ronald Britton (2015) under the name *psychic atopia*.

The term *atopia* derives from the Greek *a-topos*, meaning "without a place" or "out of place." Applied to the psyche, *psychic atopia* describes a condition in which the individual lives without a stable mental locus, or without a sense of belonging to their own psychic world. Britton observes *psychic atopia* in patients who exhibit psychotic or borderline functioning, where the sense of reality is unstable, and distinctions between self and other, between reality and fantasy, are blurred or collapsed. The mind is not capable of containing thoughts and reflecting on them. In my opinion, *psychic atopia*, a mental state lacking a stable psychic "place" where thoughts, identity, and relationships can be represented, is equivalent to *psychic withdrawal*, as I will attempt to describe it.

Meltzer (1979) makes a similar observation when he notes how the world constructed by Schreber has no anchorage in reality: suspended, elusive, it cannot be located in any precise place. It is a universe that sustains itself, devoid of coordinates that might ground it.

***Attention and Interpretation* (1970)**

In this work Bion offers us a powerful image to convey the vastness in which the psychotic patient loses both himself and his thought. It is like surgical shock: the capillaries dilate to such an extent that the patient risks bleeding to death into his own tissues.

Mental space becomes so vast that the patient feels emotion flows only to drain away into immensity. For this very reason, since there is no space delimited by coordinates, one statement remains split from another, so that contradictory elements may coexist simultaneously.

Bion reports a clinical example. A patient had once said that he could not buy any ice cream; six months later he repeated that he could not buy ice cream, and three days later he declared that it was no longer possible to buy ice cream because none remained. For Bion, "ice cream" was associatively linked to "I scream."

He formulates his interpretation as follows: the patient had been attached to his object, a good breast (he liked ice cream); he had then attacked it, perhaps literally biting it, and the bond was subsequently connoted by an "I scream." The elements of this narrative—the good breast, ice cream, envy, the bite, and the scream—were dispersed and projected into an unlimited space: no longer inhabit the same narrative space but have been expelled into an unbounded elsewhere.

Beyond this clinical example, it remains true that in the psychotic state, since no defined space or time exists, everything—every object and every individual—can be what it is, but also its opposite.

This is, in my view, a crucial turning point for the therapeutic approach to a psychotic patient highlighted by Bion. He notes that in the session the analyst can witness the transformations that the patient enacts starting from an original fact. The analyst's task, then, is not simply to interpret delusion as defense or evacuation, but to adopt a reconstructive position.

Accordingly, he must distinguish two temporalities: an observational time, in which the transformations are received as they appear, and a deductive time, in which one works to reconstruct the reality that has been distorted.

I believe this observation opens the way to a significant and necessary mode of working with the psychotic patient: not limiting oneself to denouncing the destructiveness of projective identification, but considering every psychotic communication as the result of a transformation which, although deforming, still preserves traces of an original psychic truth.

This position, intuited by Bion, departs from an approach that merely unmasks the psychotic operation, and instead places at the center the dialogue with the patient's healthy part, in order to explore together the effects that the psychotic part produces upon his mind.

In this sense, hallucination is not to be understood solely as flight or catastrophic dissolution, but as a transformation that, while annihilating space and time, nonetheless leaves visible the imprint of a psychic truth awaiting reconstruction. It is in this shared work, between observation and deduction, that one glimpses the possibility of restoring to the patient a livable mental space—not infinite and without coordinates, but once again inhabitable.

I believe it is important, at this point, to distinguish between *consciousness* and *awareness*, two concepts often considered equivalent.

Consciousness refers to the capacity to register, store, and recall a psychic event, whereas awareness concerns the meaning and understanding of that event, and is connected to the presence or absence of the intuitive function and to the capacity for self-observation.

A patient may be conscious yet unaware, in the sense that, as Bion remarks, there exist "thoughts without a thinker"; the psychotic patient, for instance, is conscious of the delusional experience and registers it, but he is unaware of its meaning.

The state of unawareness, deriving from the impossibility of employing the intuitive function, is markedly accentuated in the psychotic process. In the psychotic state, conditions emerge that are antithetical to the analytic method itself, since the latter is grounded in the possibility of new acquisitions at the level of awareness through associative work originating from unconscious intuitive processes.

On the contrary, psychopathological constructions—sometimes perverse or psychotic—distort the perception of psychic reality to the point of destroying it, creating a perceptual world antagonistic to the emotional dimension of psychic reality.

As Freud had emphasized—and as Bion reminds us—we possess an organ of consciousness capable of apprehending psychic reality. Within certain limits, we may manipulate and alter this organ, as occurs in all defensive processes. The manipulation of the organs of psychic perception may reach extreme levels, up to the creation of special worlds in which the patient remains trapped—for instance, states of sexualized well-being, perverse pleasure, or delusional psychic reality.

The psychotic patient does not employ the intuition inherent to thinking, reasoning, and scientific inquiry, which makes use of epistemic doubt, but proceeds through *illuminations* and discovers indubitable truths that suddenly appear in his mind. Knowledge through illumination is a direct form of knowing obtained without the mediation of experience, but solely by the power of the mind that creates it.

A psychotic patient whom I treated for many years told me that his delusion originated from deep within his viscera—as an intuition that overwhelmed both body and mind—something that could neither be anticipated nor contained. This intuition through illumination cannot be shared with the rest of the human community, yet the patient is not disturbed by this fact; on the contrary, he considers it a confirmation of his superiority: while the world remains in darkness, he is illuminated—and this affords him an intense pleasure.

Chapter 7

Dream and Delusion

In Bion, the unconscious loses the ontic connotation assigned to it by Freud and Melanie Klein: it is conceived not as a repository of repressed contents but as a function of the mind.

For Bion, the antithesis is not between repression (Freud) or the split unconscious (Klein) and consciousness, but rather between waking and sleeping, between what is and is not conscious at the level of awareness. The unconscious functions as a metabolizer of psychic experience, and if it does not function satisfactorily, the mind is unable to produce thoughts.

The contact-barrier and the alpha-function serve to free the mind from an excess of sensory stimuli. Dreaming constitutes the modus operandi of the psyche even in waking life: its function is to establish the contact-barrier through which beta-elements are transformed into alpha-elements and sensations become emotions.

The concept of repression is thus replaced by that of a semi-permeable membrane, a kind of unconscious organ of consciousness, which allows for the elaboration and apprehension of the world and of emotions.

This explains why a patient may be alert and lucid, and yet at the same time unaware: there can exist thoughts which fail to find an Ego capable of receiving them. In psychosis, this occurs because the alpha-function is gravely compromised: thoughts are neither retained nor transformed, but remain as fragments that drift without taking root.

Thoughts Without a Thinker

In psychotic states, thoughts lack a thinker due to the damage sustained by the alpha function. Preverbal unconscious material must be constantly subjected to the work of dreaming, which operates outside of consciousness. For Bion, "thinking" coincides with the capacity to "dream": without the ability to dream, the mind cannot think, and without the possibility of thinking, emotional experience cannot be lived.

Dreams, like the unconscious itself, are both intrapsychic and interrelational communications, rather than constructions to be interpreted. Through

DOI: 10.4324/9781003765363-8

dreaming, the unconscious provides fresh reserves of symbols and images that transform sensory experience into thought.

Unconscious material, still devoid of words and symbolic form, must constantly be subjected to the work of dreaming. It is this process—sustained by the contact-barrier, by the alpha-function, and by the transformation of beta-elements into alpha-elements—that enables the mind to elaborate what would otherwise remain inert or chaotic.

Applying this perspective to psychosis highlights a crucial point: destructiveness alone does not account for the psychotic condition. The central issue is rather that the patient is unable to think, incapable of generating the thoughts of dreaming. In psychosis, the components of unconscious functioning fail to operate: the alpha-function is absent or gravely impaired, and with it the capacity to transform sensory experience into thought collapses.

In the non-psychotic mind, by contrast, the perception of reality is continually converted into dream, and from this ceaseless work subjectivity itself emerges. Dreaming, therefore, is not a luxury of the mind but the very process that founds inner experience and makes thinking possible.

Whereas neurosis stems from a disharmonious functioning of the dynamic unconscious, psychosis originates from a profound alteration of the mental apparatus devoted to symbolizing emotions and sustaining the function of thought.

During the psychotic phase, the psychotic part of the personality blocks unconscious awareness, annihilating its capacity for intrapsychic and relational communication.

In Bion's theoretical framework, psychosis is conceived as the consequence of a failure within the unconscious apparatus responsible for emotional processing. However, it should be noted that it is not, as one might infer from Bion's account, a matter of an intact apparatus that suddenly collapses; rather, it appears from the outset as damaged and vulnerable. The persistent activity of the psychotic nucleus progressively erodes this apparatus, eventually obstructing any access to the intuitive dimension of the mind.

The Awareness

The collapse of the alpha function produces radical consequences: the patient loses the capacity for self-observation, becomes unable to access his or her own mental and emotional processes, and is deprived of the possibility of transforming sensory experiences into thoughts. In this condition, the unconscious no longer functions as a symbolic matrix but becomes "blinded," ceasing to perform its metabolic function.

For the analyst, this constitutes one of the most formidable obstacles: the psychotic patient is not simply unaware but *deprived of the very faculty of awareness*, since the unconscious functions that should process experience have been neutralized.

Unlike in neurosis—where emotional truth is repressed but not annihilated, remaining unconsciously preserved—in psychosis there is a direct break-up of the function of unconscious thinking.

Learning from experience is demolished, and meaning, instead of being safeguarded within the unconscious, is dissolved. The result is that the patient no longer has a "functioning" unconscious to which the analyst can appeal, but rather a devastated unconscious, incapable of generating dreams or symbolic thoughts.

From this void emerges an increasing dependence on an omnipotent internal system. Such a system is a parasitic construction of the mind that replaces and colonizes vital unconscious activity. It seemingly provides coherence and protection, but in reality it paralyzes thought and prevents any possibility of emotional elaboration.

Dreaming

Bion conceives of dreaming not as a circumscribed functional regression aimed at recovering repressed contents, but as a primary psychic process intrinsically devoted to the generation of thought.

Whereas for Freud the dream constituted the distorted representation of an already pre-existing unconscious meaning, for Bion it is configured as a transformative device oriented toward the production of new meaning, arising from the elaboration of the perception of emotional experience. For such perceptions to become usable within dream formation, they must acquire the quality of thought—that is, they must be transformed through the alpha function.

When this function is impaired, beta-elements remain in a raw state, without any possibility of metabolization: untransformed emotions thus present themselves as concrete sensory objects, non-symbolizable, leaving the subject incapable of dreaming and, therefore, of thinking experience.

From this perspective, the dream constitutes the royal road to the unconscious, offering evidence of the functioning of the alpha-screen and the contact-barrier. It is through these devices that the registers of psychic life can be distinguished and held in communication.

When, however, the contact-barrier is destroyed and replaced by the beta-screen, one observes a collapse of psychic functions: the capacity to discriminate between conscious and unconscious, to implement repression, to preserve mnemonic traces, and to exercise thought activity is lost. In such a clinical configuration, the subject consequently finds himself unable to produce dreams, deprived of the transformative function they carry.

Grotstein (1981), analyzed by Bion, highlights a decisive function of the dream: that of rendering psychic life thinkable and observable. For this to be possible, the presence of an internal observer must endure within the mind—an invisible yet vigilant witness, capable of noting the dream's plot, verifying its coherence, and granting validity to the implicit messages it contains.

Psychosis, by disturbing the structure and cohesion of the mental apparatus, signals the collapse of this function. The "dreamer who dreams" and the "dreamer who understands" together constitute a psychic unity that ensures the continuity of the sense of personal identity, constantly integrating emotional experience and attributing meaning to it.

The "dreamer who understands the dream" represents the capacity to receive and transform unconscious material, a function rooted in the experience of an internalized maternal container. It is this function that allows the dream to become a space of elaboration and an opening toward a possible solution.

If, however, the internal object is experienced as damaged or unreliable, the dream loses its transformative value and reverses into a persecutory experience: no longer a space of meaning, but a hostile oracle.

Under such conditions, the dream assumes the form of a psychotic experience, dominated by the refusal of knowledge (–K) and by hallucinatory drift.

One of the greatest difficulties in the analysis of dreams within the psychotic field lies precisely in the absence, in the patient, of that internal function of the "dreamer who understands the dream." Without this presence, the dream becomes undecipherable: it is no longer the product of a dialogue between the one who dreams and the one who elaborates, but is reduced to a raw sensory fragment, a testimony of mental collapse and of the loss of the mind's transformative capacity.

The destruction of the alpha function, as observed by Bion, prevents psychic experience from being deposited in unconscious memory and transformed into thinkable elements. In psychoses, dreams fail to accomplish their symbolizing function: they appear as movements struggling to emerge from chaos toward a possible attribution of meaning, but destined to remain sterile, deprived of the transformation that allows thought to take shape.

In his early work (1967), Bion had already noted that dreams in the psychotic state tend to assume a merely evacuative function: discharges of unprocessed emotions, closer to a defensive maneuver than to a genuine process of thinkability.

According to Bion, psychosis is not a dream but its very opposite. Not only are dream and psychosis not coincident, but the dreams produced in the psychotic state cannot be considered authentic dreams, even though they may assume the appearance of such. They are configured rather as concrete events, or as acts of evacuation of parts of the self, rather than as outcomes of a symbolic process.

For a dream to be defined as such, the alpha function is indispensable, since it allows the transformation of emotional experience into a representable form. In psychotic patients, however, this function is impaired: there is no internal mental space capable of containing and transforming sensory impressions, and consequently what manifests itself as a "dream" does not derive from genuine dream-work.

In this condition, dream productions no longer respond to the classical rules of the Freudian unconscious: there is neither censorship nor a latent content to which the manifest content may refer. To speak of a "psychotic unconscious" is therefore inappropriate, for the absence of dream-work prevents the formation of representations and the symbolization necessary for the very thinkability of the unconscious.

For thought to take form, an internal apparatus capable of containing it must exist. When this container is absent, awareness of what occurs in the mind is also lost.

Meltzer pursued this line of thought, exploring the ways in which the dream attempts to give symbolic form to emotional experience, transforming it into psychic truth. He describes how, at times, the dream succeeds in finding an adequate representation, while at other times it fails: it is then that the psychopathology of dreaming manifests itself. In such cases, the dream loses its symbolic function and translates into hallucinations or delusions, which, like lies, are nothing more than distorted representations of emotional experience—unfinished attempts to confer meaning upon it.

Yet, despite their fragmentary nature and apparent lack of sense, the dreams of psychotic patients may at times constitute an embryonic construction of an internal space, representing a first and fragile attempt at psychic communication. If the psychopathology of the dreaming process coincides with the distortion of thought and with the formation of hallucinations or delusions, dream productions may nonetheless reveal precious signs of the origins of such transformation.

The Delusional Dream

In my own clinical experience, I have observed that certain dreams, within the psychotic process, assume a particular significance: they appear to constitute a language through which the patient seeks to describe the mental states that characterize his or her psychosis.

In this sense, the dream may become an instrument that enables both patient and analyst to intuit and at times anticipate the quality of the psychotic transformation, or—more rarely and with greater difficulty—to outline a possible way out.

In some cases, dreams represent an attempt to render delusional contents assimilable: a kind of "dreaming the psychosis," in order to be able to look at it and begin to understand it.

Not infrequently, psychotic patients encounter great difficulty in making associations to their dreams. Dreams are experienced as alien, threatening, or incomprehensible, often arousing surprise or fear in the face of such disturbing images.

Some of these dreams, however, prove to be intimately intertwined with the psychotic condition, to the point of describing it from within: precisely for this reason, they can become invaluable material in analytic work (De Masi, 2006).

In fact, in many cases the "dreams" of psychotic patients coincide with hallucinatory or delusional constructions. Therefore, there is no metaphorical language proper to dream-work, but rather the concreteness of hallucinatory representation. These productions in fact constitute delusional reality in tangible form: the patient cannot comprehend them, even when they appear with extreme vividness.

One patient, who had gone through a psychotic episode and had been in analysis for several months following a phase of apparent remission, recounted the following dream:

> I am driving my car along a narrow road. I feel surprisingly at ease, which somewhat surprises me. At a certain point I decide not to follow the road signs anymore and realize that I am driving against traffic. This frightens me, but also excites me. I think that perhaps I should take driving lessons, but then I decide that it is not necessary, that I can continue as I am. In the end, I feel very anxious, I lose control of the car, and I find myself in a desolate land—a Martian-like landscape, scattered with cactus-like plants. I feel very alone.

This dream, situated at the boundary between dream elaboration and delusional material, seems to express from within the psychotic experience: the loss of orientation, the exhilarating transgression of rules, the sudden slide into an alien and hostile landscape. Here the dream is not only narration but a window opened onto the quality of the patient's psychic life.

The dream can be interpreted as a signal of the patient's risk of becoming trapped in the psychotic part of her mind, represented by an excited and transgressive state that drives her to defy the rules of traffic. The mixture of fear and excitement accurately reflects her internal conflict. There is a vague awareness of being guided by a dangerous and rebellious part of herself—as is evident in the thought of taking driving lessons—yet this awareness is ultimately dismissed, and the patient continues along the same path.

In the dream, the psychotic part gains dominance and drags the patient into an arid, desert-like land, a place devoid of human ties and of possibilities for exchange. With particular vividness, this scene illustrates the functioning of the psychotic part, offering the analyst a valuable tool for detecting signals of a possible recrudescence of crisis.

The dream sequence shows how the patient experiences her healthy part—represented by orderly driving, respectful of shared rules—as a sterile and meaningless routine. It is precisely this sense of emptiness that opens the way to the seduction of the psychotic part, which is instead felt as exciting and vital.

Unlike the neurotic patient, who fears madness and resists it, the psychotic patient allows himself to be drawn to its call: the illusory promise of omnipotence. It is this fascination that dulls the fear of madness and propels him into a dangerous mental state, where the euphoria of omnipotence prepares the ground for collapse.

Aldo, a young psychotic patient, once told me he had dreamed of a church with a tennis court. At the time he reported this dream he was feeling better and had recently resumed playing tennis, a sport he had loved in his teens.

Aldo offered no associations to the dream, and I initially found myself unable to say anything useful about it. In subsequent sessions he spoke repeatedly about the pleasure he derived from playing and even mentioned entering a tournament organized by his club.

Only later did it become apparent that he had become completely and delusionally identified with the then world champion, John McEnroe. An episode of enacted delusional behavior in his parish church subsequently revealed that he also saw himself as a reincarnation of Jesus Christ.

Only then did the communicative value of Aldo's "dream" become intelligible: it had concretely fused two strands of a grandiose delusion—sport (the tennis court / McEnroe) and mysticism (the church / Christ).

Aldo had presented the dream without associations and, in a session, produced what amounted to a hallucination; yet at the time it was impossible to work through it because I remained convinced that the "dream" symbolized something else to be interpreted. In this case, the "dream" and its content do not refer to the metaphorical discourse of dream-work, but to the concrete nature of the delusion construction; the dream image is communicating the construction of a new sensory reality, which in essence is different from the symbolic nature of dreams.

Emerging from the megalomaniac state signaled by that initial dream, he later reported another dream that could be read as representing the psychotic transformation and persecutory guilt.

In this later dream he had been invited to the home of an analyst couple who let him climb into their double bed. There he became aroused, performing a series of twisting and turning movements that terminated in a blissful state of pleasure. Then the figures of his parents appeared, faint and distant. Finally he found himself surrounded by deformed basset hounds with their heads wrenched back, who accused him of being responsible for their deformity.

This time Aldo felt that the small deformed animals in the dream represented parts of himself—little selves. The scene had visualized the masturbatory pleasure that underlay the onset of his delusion of omnipotence; but now he also grasped the destructive quality of that process on himself—how it had caused psychic damage and weakened both the analyst and his parents.

In delusions, something paradoxical occurs regarding the dream: as opposed to being considered as mysterious with a meaning to discover, the delusion is frightening in that its meaning, whether exciting or persecutory, is concrete. If dreams proper serve to make *unconscious awareness* in each of us explicit, such awareness is absent in these patients.

It can therefore be assumed that without the apparatus for thinking thoughts, dreams are meaningless and disconnected from each other. To put it another way, in severe pathologies the possibility to think and dream is absent because there is no observing ego (the thinker or the narrator).

This poses an important question for analytic therapy: how can an observer capable of thinking thoughts be developed? And what prevented its development in the first place?

It seems that in some patients the emotional field has not had the opportunity to develop adequately. The observer who understands the dream has the function of understanding psychic reality, that is, our emotional reality. However, this operation is possible when the emotional field is active and the dynamic unconscious, after repressing unbearable emotional states, keeps them registered in unconscious memory.

The value of such clinical material lies in the fact that dreams not only anticipate the contents of psychosis but also describe with precision its internal functioning: they show the seductive and disorienting action of the psychotic part, capable of destabilizing and destroying the subject's mental health.

By restoring to the patient the meaning of the dream and clarifying how her psychotic part operates the analyst can establish a connection with the healthy part, which appears subordinated and intimidated by the psychotic part.

This aspect is crucial, because, as Bion emphasized, the failure to recognize the signals of the psychotic part's action within analytic communication increases the risk of a delusional collapse.

The analyst who succeeds in perceiving the seductive or intimidating effect exerted by the psychotic part on the healthy part can help the patient escape this trap. Conversely, when the delusional dream is not understood, the patient experiences a sense of triumph that pushes him even further into psychotic colonization.

It must not be forgotten that therapists can easily be deceived: many patients conceal their delusional experiences and allow only an apparently coherent communication to emerge. In such cases, the risk is to remain confined to the explicit content, without recognizing the psychotic processes operating in depth. Insight then arrives too late, when psychosis has already taken hold and the patient realizes that he has become trapped in the reality he himself has constructed.

Some psychotic dreams provide direct access to the core of the delusional transformation, yet they do not necessarily promote an immediate increase in self-awareness: the patient's conscious Ego for a long time remains subordinated and colonized by the delusional organization.

It is therefore essential to work persistently on dreams that stage the psychotic process and display the patient's investment in it. The dream thus becomes not only a testimony of the psychotic process, but also an opportunity to explore the internal dynamic between attraction and submission.

If delusion may be conceived as an "omnipotent dream" that supplants psychic reality, the psychotic dream—which evidences the pressure of delusion in the very act of colonizing the Ego—acquires diagnostic and therapeutic value. It signals the catastrophic risk inherent in the psychotic process and offers the analyst a point of intervention aimed at loosening the seductive yet threatening hold of delusion.

The theoretical framework elaborated by Bion on the nature and function of dreaming enables us to consider certain psychotic dreams as instruments for analytic work. Clinical contributions by Meltzer, Grotstein, and others, as well as the observations reported here, are indebted to Bion's distinction between psychotic and non-psychotic parts of the personality and to his theory of thinking.

The concrete, a-symbolic quality of psychotic dreams reflects the absence of alpha-function: some dreams are reduced to primitive sensory sequences or degenerate into hallucinations. Consequently, the boundary between oneiric experience and lived reality becomes indeterminate, leaving the patient unable to discriminate between the two.

Bion emphasized that in psychotic states repression is not operative and the dynamic unconscious does not function in classical terms.

Nevertheless, as treatment progresses, certain dreams reveal the seductive strategies of the psychotic part over the non-psychotic part, operating through illusory promises of omnipotence, triumph, and pleasure—psychic mirages that usurp contact with reality.

Only in more advanced phases of the analysis do dreams begin to contain symbolic configurations, thereby opening the way to dynamic interpretation.

Such dreams testify to the gradual capacity of the non-psychotic part of the personality to employ unconscious functions essential to personality development.

Chapter 8

A Multi-Handed Development

It is possible to distinguish two major orientations in the development of Bion's conceptualization of psychosis.

In the initial phase of his work, Bion is fully situated within the Kleinian framework, placing at the center of his reading the destructive drive and projective identification as constitutive nuclei of the psychotic experience.

Even when he introduces original elements—such as the distinction between the healthy part and the psychotic part of the personality—the latter is described as an intrinsically destructive drive configuration, one that hates reality and attacks the apparatus of knowledge.

This perspective, however, does not yet allow him to conceive of psychosis as a disturbance of the very functioning of the mind, as will instead occur in the second phase of his theoretical–clinical inquiry.

Despite his numerous attempts, even in the second part of his work, Bion never arrives at a fully elaborated vision of the psychotic part which may become evident during the analytic process. It is plausible that the epistemological method he privileged in his later period may have, at least in part, diverted him from the direct clinical observation of the patient that had characterized his earlier research.

Although he acknowledged that even in the confused or delusional patient a healthy nucleus always persists, Bion does not develop an in-depth analysis of either the dynamic or the shifting equilibrium between the two parts, nor does he fully highlight the role that the healthy part may assume in the course of therapy when confronted with psychotic functioning.

He does not describe in detail the ways in which the psychotic part operates, nor does he emphasize its seductive and corrupting power over the healthy part, focusing instead on the problem of the transformation of sensory elements into thoughts.

Bion's early clinical writings also tend to focus on the destructive effects of psychotic action—attacks on linking, distortions of reality, omnipotent arrogance—without fully grasping the unstable and fragile equilibrium between the healthy and the psychotic part.

DOI: 10.4324/9781003765363-9

Rather than conceiving of a progressive colonization of the healthy part by the psychotic part, Bion seems to imagine a sharp split that separates and rigidly maintains them apart.

Bion's theory of the attack on perceptual function, of primal envy, and of the attack on the analyst, while highly fertile, nevertheless proves insufficient to account for the nature of the power that the psychotic part exerts over the patient, progressively leading him to an open crisis.

It is true that psychotic illness entails the destruction of the capacity to think, to live emotions, and to construct a sense of identity; what remains to be clarified, however, are the pathways through which such transformation unfolds.

In my view, it is not a matter of direct and explicit aggression—as occurs in perversions—but rather of a sophisticated, insidious, and deceptive process that subtly alters perceptions and the contact with reality.

The emphasis Bion had placed on the destructive action of the psychotic part loses centrality once he elaborates his theory of thought.

Destructiveness is no longer conceived as a kind of "original sin" that looms over the patient throughout his existence; rather, the fundamental defect is traced back to a deficiency of the function of thought, indispensable for accessing knowledge of reality and fostering psychic development.

Although never fully embracing this position, Bion also identifies a relational origin of this deficit. The child acquires knowledge and a sense of his own emotions through contact with the mother's mind. If the latter is unable to exercise a function of containment and elaboration, a deficit of the alpha function ensues.

In the absence of this symbolizing capacity, unprocessed mental products remain at a sensory level and are treated as beta-elements, devoid of psychic integration.

From this perspective, the aim of therapy takes shape as a transformative process: the passage from sensory (beta) elements to psychic (alpha) elements, which enables the patient to develop intuitive functions and a progressive awareness of self and reality.

The Work of the Psychotic Part

Among Bion's contemporaries, Rosenfeld appears more attentive in grasping the dynamic between the psychotic part and the healthy part in the analytic field. He observes that, once captured by the psychotic part, the patient perceives himself as immersed in a dimension that is separate and impermeable with respect to the external world.

The delusional withdrawal generates in him the conviction that he can gain access to an absolute pleasure, within a condition of total anarchy. Precisely because of this seductive promise, the delusional nucleus exerts a powerful attraction on the healthy parts of the personality, progressively inducing them to abandon the world of relationships and adhere to the psychotic logic.

He writes:

> the narcissistic psychotic part of the self exerts its power and superiority over life and the analyst, standing for reality, by trying to lure the dependent self into a psychotic omnipotent dream state which results in the patient losing his sense of reality and his capacity for thinking. In fact there is a danger of an acute psychotic state if the dependent part of the patient, which is the sanest part of his personality, is persuaded to turn away from the external world and give itself up entirely to the domination of the psychotic delusional structure.
>
> (Rosenfeld, 1971, p. 175)

A clinical observation by Fromm-Reichmann clearly illustrates this dynamic: one of her psychotic patients, during a session, managed to speak to her about the delusional reality in which she lived. At the following session, however, she was unable to appear, having been threatened with death by the psychotic part for having revealed to the analyst their secret pact.

It is well known how complex it is to escape from the psychotic world. If, as Rosenfeld states, the psychotic part acts as a delinquent-mafia-like structure, it becomes evident that it will intensify its attacks as the patient attempts to free himself from its domination, alternating strategies of terror and seduction.

In this way it becomes clear how research on psychosis in Bion and Rosenfeld proceeds in part in parallel and in part diverging. Bion, through his theory of thought, emphasizes the patient's incapacity to transform sensory impressions into thought; Rosenfeld, instead, opens the way to a clinical and dynamic conception of the relation between the two parts of the personality, underlining their conflict and mutual attraction.

These two perspectives, though seemingly divergent, can find a possible integration if one considers the psychotic state in its full complexity. Psychotic functioning of the mind must in fact be imagined as a developmental trajectory that originates in childhood. Some children, predisposed to this modality, tend progressively to withdraw into a sensory reality that eventually replaces relational thought.

The outcome is a paradoxical coexistence of two realities, the sensory and the psychic, which proceed in parallel: what is real for one part of the mind is not so for the other.

Bion had a decisive intuition on this point when he affirmed that the psychotic patient cannot resort to repression, but must rely exclusively on projective identification. This modality, founded on expulsion, annuls awareness and obstructs the activation of the alpha function, reducing thought to a sequence of sensory elements incapable of entering the unconscious and of becoming thinkable.

In my opinion, in the case of psychosis, the attack on consciousness—on which Bion insisted in his early clinical writings—does not occur through a direct assault on linking, but rather through the very exclusion of awareness of what is happening, consequent to the use of the mind in a purely sensory modality.

It concerns the creation, in childhood, of a world in which the presence of reality is annulled in favor of a dimension where frustration, waiting, and doubt no longer exist, and where imagination replaces reality and assumes its very features.

Winnicott described an infantile psychic withdrawal (although he did not name it in these terms) in relation to a clinical case of primary dissociation. He defines this phenomenon as a retreat into a dissociated state of fantasies—a defensive mechanism against the oppressive sensation of non-existence.

Although in his writings Winnicott often emphasizes the vital and creative aspects of fantasy, on the contrary in this paper he highlights its defensive value, showing how it may take the form of a psychic withdrawal from reality. In this dissociative state, many things may happen, yet in fact nothing truly authentic occurs: the subject does not experience his or her existence as that of a complete human being.

By contrast, when fantasy supports development, it gradually transforms—through processes of integration and personalization—into the capacity to imagine, which is intimately connected to both dreaming and reality.

Psychic Retreats

In his stimulating volume *Psychic Retreats* (1993), John Steiner describes a wide range of mechanisms through which the subject creates psychic states that protect against anxiety and pain. These are mental spaces into which the patient withdraws after breaking off contact with the analyst.

Psychic retreat—constructed as a defense both against schizoid–paranoid and against depressive anxiety—may assume very different forms: from refuge in a romantic, fairytale world where everything appears idealized, to a masturbatory withdrawal marked by pornographic excitement. According to Steiner, these pathological personality organizations function as a kind of drug for an ego damaged by the assaults of reality and incapable of genuine reparative processes.

While such a pathological organization serves the function of defending against anxiety, it also protects the subject from depressive pain, thereby enabling him to avoid the experience of loss. The patient idealizes the delusional world and presents it as a pleasant refuge, a sanctuary against the psychotic terror of disintegration and annihilation.

As Steiner observes, even when the patient recognizes that the constructed retreat is a mad, cruel, and persecutory reality, it still remains preferable to the fear and pain experienced in the external world.

In my view (De Masi, 2006, 2020), the construction of retreat originates in childhood, when the structuring relationship with the parental mind fails for various reasons. Once the child takes refuge in this inner world, he becomes independent of adults and ceases to learn from emotional experience.

The retreat appears as a space populated by pleasurable and gratifying sensations, in which the child cultivates an illusion of power that provides him with a state of superiority and self-sufficiency, thereby eliminating the need to depend on external human objects.

The mind constructs this retreat through its own sensory and imaginative functions, effectively withdrawing it from the dynamic unconscious and from the symbolic dimension.

Primitive infantile retreat hinders the development of personality and inhibits the growth of subjective psychic reality; its psychopathological structure may be conceptualized as the psychotic part of the personality.

The features of pre-psychotic personality—marked by a lack of emotional involvement, of curiosity, and of the capacity to form meaningful relationships—may be regarded as epiphenomena of a mind transformed by retreat.

In this mental state, the mind functions predominantly as a sensory organ: sensory data replace psychic data, erasing intuitive, perceptive, and relational functions.

Although this is not the only process contributing to the development of illness, it represents one of the primary pathways through which the mind both develops and, at the same time, internalizes pathology.

Psychic retreat fosters the emergence of the psychotic part of the personality, which constructs an alternative reality founded upon sensory bases.

This psychotic reality may coexist for a long time with the healthy part of the mind, manifesting clinically only at the moment of psychotic breakdown.

The extreme anxiety accompanying psychosis is released when the predominance of the psychotic part over the healthy part reaches its peak: at that point the patient feels lost, unable to find the path back to reality.

The psychotic patient may live for years in his own ivory tower, viewing the world exclusively through his projections. Lacking a sense of separateness between self and other, or between self and the surrounding world, he does not raise questions about what does not belong to him and what he does not know. As Bion repeatedly emphasized, he does not learn from experience.

For there to be an experience of the other, it is necessary to question our selves, to recognize the differences that constitute us as separate individuals. But the mode of functioning based on sensory projections, in which the psychotic remains imprisoned, does not permit the perception of difference. Thus he formulates no questions, cultivates no curiosity, discovers nothing: sensory thinking nourishes him in a self-referential manner, without recourse to the external world.

My clinical experience has led me to observe with wonder how to observe how, after years of analytic work, the psychotic patient who manages to emerge from retreat gradually discovers what for others is the natural process of thought: listening to the other, perceiving one's own emotions and deriving from them an indication of the content of communication; formulating hypotheses about the other's reality as distinct from oneself; and finally grasping the meaning of what has occurred in the relationship.

Chapter 9

A Consideration on the Present

The period between the 1950s and 1970s, marked by the writings of Bion, Rosenfeld, and Segal, opened unprecedented perspectives in the analytic work with psychotic patients. This renewed focus on psychosis seemed to represent a genuine revolutionary development in the understanding of severe mental disorders.

From a contemporary standpoint, however, it becomes clear that the application of Kleinian theory—including the fundamental theoretical and clinical contributions of Bion—has not evolved into an equally fertile and linear clinical practice, when compared to what the theory seemed to promise.

Surveying the psychoanalytic literature, one can easily observe how the interest in the treatment of psychotic patients within the Kleinian framework has progressively diminished. What is striking, moreover, is the limited discussion—both within and outside the Kleinian group—regarding the reasons for this decline. In fact, the concepts elaborated by Melanie Klein, and later by Bion, did not translate directly into therapeutic interventions of consistent efficacy with psychotic patients.

Despite the broadening of theoretical horizons brought about by Klein and the post-Kleinians, the corresponding—and much anticipated—progress in clinical outcomes has not occurred.

This may also account for the reduction, in recent decades, of analytic publications devoted to clinical work with psychotic patients. As I have already suggested—and as I shall develop further—there remain intrinsically complex knots within the treatment of psychotic processes that still await resolution.

In my view, the difficulty does not reside solely in the challenge of tolerating the depressive position, as emphasized by Bion, Segal, and Rosenfeld.

What I have observed, rather, is that when these patients show improvement after a prolonged stay in the psychotic state, they often abandon the arduous path of acquiring the psychic and emotional capacities necessary for engaging in relationships.

Instead, they seem to prefer returning to the denial of reality and to the delusional state. Evidently, the delusional experience becomes deeply embedded within the psyche and appears to resist every attempt at transformation.

DOI: 10.4324/9781003765363-10

As Meg Harris Williams writes, Donald Meltzer explicitly addressed the difficulty of treating psychotic patients, acknowledging the immense challenges inherent in such treatment:

> Meltzer… worked for many years with severely ill and schizophrenic patients but said that it was only possible to work with their non-delusional parts, not with the large area of the personality that had succumbed to delusion. In terms of internal geography, he regarded extreme projective or adhesive identification as bringing the personality to a kind of tipping-point beyond which it became lost to help and retrieval.
>
> (Harris Williams, 2022, p. 68)

Another testimony comes from John Steiner, who, on the occasion of the webinar presentation of a book in his honor, *The Allure of Psychic Retreats* (edited by Heinz Weiss), on 7 December 2024 (https://vimeo.com/1038501737), stated that, on the basis of the positive experiences described by the analysts in his group, he had tried unsuccessfully to treat some psychotic cases and had to give up with great bitterness.

This explicit recognition by Meltzer and Steiner reflects a broader acknowledgment within the psychoanalytic community of the limitations and difficulties involved in treating psychotic patients, and the need for the development of new strategies and techniques suited to their particular psychological needs.

One of the reasons that led me to write this book is the conviction that today there exists the concrete risk that Bion's invaluable insights into psychosis may be progressively forgotten: destined to remain as theoretical formulations, without finding any real integration into clinical practice.

Bion's iconic style and his extraordinary capacity to grasp what is not immediately visible explain, at least in part, the posthumous success of his ideas. Nevertheless, concepts such as the "attack on linking," the "psychotic part of the personality," or the "alpha function," although they have entered common usage, rarely seem to translate into an authentic clinical method capable of keeping alive the original spirit of his intuitions.

The treatment of psychotic patients is undoubtedly long, complex, and difficult, but it can become fruitful if the analyst succeeds in adopting the right position. We must not forget the infinite heuristic power of psychoanalysis: before us opens a mind that speaks an unknown language, and the task of the analyst is to learn how to decipher it.

Starting from the concepts deriving from the theory of thought, we must accept that it is not possible to use the usual interpretative language, since, in the absence of the alpha function, there is no dynamic unconscious nor the capacity to understand and introject the analyst's words. Rather, we find ourselves in a world without time and without space, in which affirmation and negation may coexist simultaneously within the same object. The analyst may be perceived as benevolent and, a moment later, as persecutory; the patient's wife may be experienced at once as a loving companion and as a murderer.

In other words, it is necessary to learn from within the functioning of the psychotic part of the personality and the universe it constructs within the patient's psyche. As Bion observed, this is a space-time continually occupied by bizarre objects and propositions, which prevent the existence of a free space-time—one not sensorially invaded, but open instead to creativity and thought.

The analyst, despite the distortions and apparent incongruities that characterize such a world, must maintain a vigilant mind, ready to register this reality, which escapes stable and constant coordinates and initially presents itself as unpredictable.

To communicate with a psychotic patient means to establish a link that allows a dialogue with his psychotic part. This process requires a profound and systematic knowledge of the origins and evolution of the illness. Analysts who work with such patients are acutely aware of the necessity of approaching them with extreme caution and sensitivity.

The psychotic individual is firmly convinced of the absolute truth of his delusion, defends it rigidly, and may perceive the analyst as an antagonist. Until the patient succeeds, through his healthy part, in developing a genuine collaboration with the analyst—one that enables him to access an introspective capacity for thought—every therapeutic perspective remains uncertain and fragile.

It is always necessary to keep one's gaze directed also toward the patient's childhood. As the patient gradually acquires awareness and develops the capacity to observe himself critically as a child, he provides, in the course of therapy, precious elements for understanding the origins of his psychotic disorder.

From this perspective, Bion does not offer sufficient tools. The child who emerges in his writings is in fact the impersonal child of the theory of thinking: a child who, in order to survive, projects intolerable sensations into the mother's mind, so that she may render them thinkable. The psychosis that transpires from Bion's texts does not assume that complex, varied, and dramatic character that we encounter in other clinical accounts; the major gain derived from Bion's writings is situated primarily at the theoretical level.

In reconstructing the childhood of several psychotic patients, it often emerges that the minds of the parents resemble those described by Bion in his theory of thinking: minds unable to decode the child's communications and therefore incapable of providing the introjections necessary to sustain the formation of an adequate identity in the child.

However, the problem does not lie solely in this lack of receptivity. Projective identification, in fact, operates in both directions, and one must also consider the reverse movement: the projections originating from the parents that are deposited in the child's mind.

In my clinical experience, I have repeatedly observed how some children destined to develop psychosis grow up with the unshakable conviction that they may become geniuses. Such certainty, far from being spontaneous, is often the effect of parental propaganda that implants within the child a delusional nucleus, exalting supposed exceptional qualities. The child, seduced by this idealization, transfers this legacy into the parallel world of withdrawal, which preserves and elaborates it in isolation from reality.

From this parallel world, the psychotic part of the personality takes shape, engaged in imposing an omnipotent desire up to the psychotic crisis—understood as the ultimate attempt to erase reality once and for all, the very reality that contradicts its grandiose presumption. Persecution, always in delusional form, appears subsequently, when responsibility for failure is attributed to powerful enemies, envious of the patient's glory and determined to obstruct it.

Chapter 10

My Vision

I first turned to the study of psychosis as an analyst nearly 40 years ago, after two decades of working as a psychiatrist in both hospital and outpatient settings. My transition into psychoanalysis carried with it the hope that the analytic framework—with its continuity and relational depth—might provide the most suitable instrument for approaching the enigmatic core of psychosis.

As I have written elsewhere (De Masi, 2006), my early attempts were far from encouraging; only gradually did I learn to listen and to understand psychotic patients in a more effective way. It quickly became clear to me that the necessary clinical competence could not be acquired in isolation. This led me to devote many years to building a discussion and supervision group with analysts working with psychotic patients, and later another group focusing on severely disturbed children.

What has always stayed with me is the impression that a single lifetime is not enough to truly understand psychosis. Insights that appear to have been gained often need to be rethought, relocated, and placed in a broader perspective.

The path requires perseverance, the capacity to tolerate frustration, and the determination not to abandon the journey even when it feels arduous or uncertain. In this sense, Bion's work and example have been for me a luminous guide—one of rigor, courage, and dedication.

Across the decades I have come to believe that I have identified certain essential elements in the origins and development of psychosis, but above all, I have learned what kind of clinical stance most effectively opens the way to a communication that can truly benefit the patient.

Among the many authors who have shaped my thinking, Bion has been the most enduring companion. Yet, while acknowledging the fruitfulness of his ideas, I have gradually distanced myself from one of his most recurrent hypotheses, shared by many within the Kleinian tradition: the view that psychosis is fueled primarily by destructiveness.

The hypothesis of the death drive undoubtedly has descriptive power. To conceive psychosis as a process of inner demolition captures well the lived experience of psychic collapse.

DOI: 10.4324/9781003765363-11

But such a perspective risks obscuring both the origins and the evolution of the disorder, pushing into the background the pathogenic role of the early environment—especially the parental environment—from which the child first learns to think. It also fails to explain why psychosis may remain latent for years and then suddenly erupt with devastating force.

By contrast, I consider Bion's second line of reflection on psychosis to be irreplaceable.

If, as he suggests, the psychotic individual is unable to make use of the alpha function and thus cannot transform sensory impressions into thought, then what has happened in the mind? What pathway has led such a person to privilege the sensory dimension, choosing to remain within it—as though it offered not only irresistible fascination but also a refuge, an alternative to the world of thought?

At a certain stage my inquiry shifted toward the study of children who, even in the earliest years of life, seemed perilously close to the psychotic universe. Since then, in my work with adults as well, I have sought to reconstruct their early histories, as well as those of patients discussed in supervision. There are indeed children who appear strikingly different from their peers: they inhabit a separate world, show little need for closeness, do not seek shared play, and seem largely uninterested in relationships with others.

An Alternative World

Some children retreat into a sensory domain, a space to be inhabited alone and at a distance from the surrounding world. The psychic universe of emotions, desires, and feelings is gradually replaced by a world of images and scenarios constructed through the sensory apparatus of the mind.

It was in this context that I introduced, in a number of publications, the concept of *sensory withdrawal*, elaborating it from John Steiner's notion of *psychic retreat* (De Masi, 2024).

A delicate and telling literary example of sensory withdrawal can be found in Dostoevsky's *White Nights*. The protagonist does not appear as an ordinary man, but as a creature who, like a tortoise, withdraws into his shell. He lives immersed in an imaginary world, in a ceaseless dream before which real life loses all significance. He desires nothing, he feels himself beyond desire itself, for he is convinced that he is the artist of his own existence, which he endlessly recreates.

In this dimension, the subject authorizes himself to believe that what he imagines is neither a mirage nor a deception, but something real. Yet this idyllic condition is not stable: even the dreamer is assailed by moments of anguish, in which he feels he has lost all contact with reality and is living only within a dream, devoid of substance.

Sensory withdrawal often originates in childhood and may be traced back to a deficit in the primary mother–infant relationship, which should have sustained psychic development.

As Bion observed, from the very first days of life the infant establishes a primordial communication with the caregiver, preceding verbal language. This early exchange—composed of the infant's implicit questions before an unknown world and the parents' emotional responses—is essential for maintaining contact with reality.

When such a process of reception and understanding is absent or insufficient, a tendency toward sensory withdrawal may emerge: the child turns inward into his own body or constructs a world of sensory fantasies that distances him from reality and protects him from emotional dependence on adults.

It has long been recognized in psychoanalysis that abnormal and maladaptive behavior arises when, during the crucial period of self-formation, the child is deprived of sensory stimulation or adequate emotional attunement.

When the infant's needs are met, by contrast, sensory gratification naturally integrates into an affective context: physical tenderness, caresses, hugs, and kisses become spontaneous relational exchanges. But what happens when this process is interrupted?

In the absence of emotional input from the caregiver, the child turns either to his own body or to a dissociated world to procure stimulation. Sensation, stripped of the relational quality born of interaction, becomes distorted. To counter the threat of psychic disintegration, the deprived child clings to elementary sensory experiences—a light, a voice, a smell—that serve as a kind of adhesive for the fragments of his personality. Alternatively, he may seek refuge in self-stimulatory behaviors or in masturbatory activities.

O'Shaughnessy (1992) describes this process with clarity, distinguishing between the child who is able to tolerate frustration by using the precursors of thought—for instance, crying until the mother intervenes to comfort him—and the less fortunate one, who instead evacuates frustration (and with it, reality) without being able to transform it. The latter does not cry, remains silent, and fixes his attention on a sensory detail: thus begins a withdrawal which, relying on perceptual channels, constructs an alternative reality—pleasant, protective, and shielding him from the relational dependency required for emotional development.

This may represent one of the pathways through which a sensory world dissociated from reality takes shape. It is important to emphasize that the process does not occur immediately, but develops gradually and, in cases that evolve toward psychosis, tends to replace the functions of intuitive thought that should have been supported by the alpha function.

In my view, this is not merely a defense against the pain of frustration, but also a choice drawn by the intrinsic fascination of the sensory world. This universe presents itself to the child as more immediate, concrete, and gratifying—a sort of refuge that alleviates anxiety and promises direct pleasure. From this perspective, sensory withdrawal should not be understood solely as the product of a failure of thought, but rather as the construction of an alternative reality that the child learns to privilege over relational reality, experienced as too uncertain and demanding.

This sensory world remains for a long time separate from reality, compelling the individual to oscillate between two dimensions. The psychopathological structure of withdrawal may persist indefinitely, tending to expand until it invades and ultimately dominates the entire personality.

Analysts working with children often observe processes that may foreshadow the development of psychosis. Children predisposed to such an outcome are frequently neglected or misunderstood by their parents, who are unable to distinguish between ordinary childhood fantasies and the construction of a world detached from reality—sometimes even mistaking it for a state of calm or serenity.

Teachers often describe these children as struggling with learning difficulties or problems in social relationships. In truth, their connection with others is merely superficial: they lead a secret, parallel life, retreating into an inner world rich in sensory experiences.

This alternative universe, inhabited by imaginary figures and at times fueled by obsessive consumption of television or digital cartoons, replaces real life. The gravest consequence of such withdrawal is that the child fails to develop a psychic apparatus (what Bion calls alpha function) capable of comprehending and elaborating psychic reality.

Even if not yet overtly ill, a child of this kind remains disconnected from self-awareness, unable to perceive the emotional reactions of others, and fearful of relational experience—an experience he neither desires, nor understands, and which ultimately frightens him.

Patients predisposed to psychosis thus inhabit two separate realities. Alongside external, everyday life, a dissociated and parallel world persists, providing stimulation and excitement. This alternative reality reduces or even abolishes the need for genuine relationships with others. Over time, withdrawal may evolve into a full-blown delusion, when the imaginary world invades the patient's mind until it is experienced as entirely real.

At this point, it is worth recalling that Melanie Klein had already noted that schizoid mechanisms may exert a deleterious effect on intellectual development, and that certain forms of mental retardation should be regarded as belonging to the category of schizophrenias (Klein, 1946).

The psychological absence of the parents, or alternatively their narcissistic intrusiveness, fosters the child's retreat into an omnipotent world. It is within this space that the delusional structure is forged, which, in time, will unfold into its grandiose and persecutory dimensions.

In my view, psychic withdrawal is not merely a protective measure against anxiety, relational emptiness, or the sense of meaninglessness. It is, above all, a place of pleasure, where the patient feels like a god, capable of creating objects and realities out of nothing. To preserve this withdrawal, however, the subject must conceal it—first from his parents and later, in analysis, from the analyst himself.

It is crucial not to underestimate the progressive and harmful effects of childhood withdrawal. Whereas play enriches the child's emotional world, sensory withdrawal stifles curiosity and traps the child within a closed, self-sufficient reality.

It is a system that seduces the patient narcissistically, attributing to him merits he does not possess and conquering him with a pleasure resembling a state of intoxication, almost drug-like.

Only at a later stage does the psychotic part reveal its destructive face, manifesting as a delinquent organization that attacks, intimidates, and threatens the healthy part of the personality.

Thus, it is not the destructive drive that primarily moves the psychotic part, but rather the force of pleasure, which guides and perverts the patient's awareness. Psychosis appears as a condition in which the mind not only fails in its task of transforming beta sensory elements into thought, but seems to produce endlessly new sensory elements.

During the psychotic state, in hallucinations and delusion the patient "sees" with the eyes of his mind, hears and perceives voices with the "ears" of his mind: an inner world populated with perceptions that for him have the same consistency as external reality.

For the psychotic mind, the problem is not merely the inability to transform sensory elements into thoughts, but the fact that it produces only sensory elements. The difficulty of the psychotic patient in symbolizing and representing may thus be understood as follows: in psychic withdrawal, which precedes the psychotic explosion, mental functioning undergoes a transformation, shifting from a psychic register to a sensory one (De Masi, 2020).

In his hypothesis on the psychopathology of psychosis, Bion did not adopt the perspective that conceives delusion as the progressive construction, beginning in childhood, of an alternative sensory world.

In "On Hallucination" (1958), describing a patient who complained of being unable to distinguish what is real from what is not, he recalls the conceptualization of the excessive use of projective identification (p. 125). The patient's inability to discern between real and imaginary results from the expulsion, through projective identification, of the function of judgment from his own mind.

Bion even went so far as to hypothesize that among the many bizarre objects generated by the excessive use of this mechanism, there might be one assimilable precisely to the faculty of judgment, which reappears in the form of a delusional manifestation. Certain delusions, according to Bion, may be considered attempts to employ such bizarre objects in the service of a therapeutic intuition. Deeper insights into the dynamics of the psychotic state derive from Bion's theory of thinking.

During the acute psychotic crisis, the mind, excited and dominated by sensory functioning, loses all control and advances unrestrained toward a catastrophe both terrifying and at the same time exhilarating. The untransformed beta-elements detonate like an atomic explosion, leaving behind a radioactive desert ready to contaminate what remains of the healthy part.

Bion's conceptualization (1957) of the psychotic part of the personality, if interpreted as imbued with a pathological sensoriality capable of distorting the perception of psychic reality, constitutes an essential point of reference for understanding the process. In cases destined for psychotic development, the crisis emerges when the sensory constructions elaborated in withdrawal succeed in conquering the entire healthy part of the personality.

Psychotic breakdown never occurs suddenly: one must assume a long, silent work of preparation over time. Just as a wooden structure may collapse abruptly because it has been progressively corroded by a colony of termites, so the psychotic collapse, though appearing sudden, is in fact the outcome of a slow, constant, and hidden process.

Meltzer emphasized, though without naming it as such, the pathogenic role of withdrawal in the development of delusion:

> We must not, in my view, lose sight of the disturbing possibility that this quiet and silent process may occur in anyone during the course of development, and that, alongside more familiar forms of development, a delusional system may simultaneously take shape, underground.
>
> (1979, p. 42)

This "quiet and motionless world" presents itself as an alternative to mental growth and to communication with the external world.

Delusion is pure sensoriality, devoid of access to representation and symbolization; it is founded upon symbolic equations (Segal, 1957), and, in my view, it is in this sense that Bion's statement concerning the inversion of the alpha function must be understood. In delusion, imagination—which under normal conditions mediates ideational or representational content—is unconsciously transformed into beta-elements, that is, into pure sensory data.

The delusional structure rests, therefore, on this peculiar capacity of the psychotic mind to convert imaginative thought into sensoriality: it cannot be integrated into dream-work, nor generate transformative psychic experiences such as fantasy or thought, since it corresponds to a non-thought, to –K described by Bion (1992).

Even outside the acute crisis, the most compromised psychic areas are those devoted to intuitive and emotional thinking: the excess of sensoriality invades and saturates the relational channels of the mind, obstructing the possibility of symbolic elaboration. Psychic experience thus loses its subjective character and is lived as a concrete, tangible, sensory world. The mind functions as if it were a perceptive organ, capable of generating alternative worlds in which to take refuge: a true psychic retreat.

And it is precisely because this alternative world is constructed by the psychotic part starting from sensory perception that it appears to the patient not as illusory, but as absolutely real and true.

The therapeutic work with the psychotic part of the personality represents only the initial phase of the analytic task. With the gradual emergence of the healthy part, which progressively succeeds in containing the psychotic aspects and in moving out of isolation, the patient nevertheless finds himself unable to face life fully. Understanding the other and experiencing emotions in a meaningful way remain, for him, extremely complex and difficult tasks. For this reason, he tends to minimize the space of confrontation with reality.

The analyst often finds himself in dialogue with a "two-dimensional" person. This derives from the fact that the patient, having lived for a long time in a psychic retreat and in an alternative reality, has never truly learned how to relate to the external world. It is as though he were a being who had lived on the moon and had no notion of what it means to inhabit the earth.

The analyst's task thus becomes that of accompanying the patient in his development and supporting him in the slow process of reclaiming a properly human dimension, and tolerating that, when faced with tasks perceived as impossible, he may regress. For this reason, the analyses of psychotic patients tend to be of very long duration. And yet, one must acknowledge that this arduous task, if pursued with constancy and perseverance, can generate a profound sense of mutual gratitude, both in the patient and in the analyst.

The Seeds of Madness

The concept of psychic retreat integrates a range of psychoanalytic observations. It elucidates the sensory concreteness of thought, grandiosity, and subsequent feelings of persecution, the absence of symbolic and intuitive mental functions, and the blurring of boundaries between the inner and outer worlds.

An author who came very close to the notion of infantile retreat as the original nucleus of a possible psychotic organization is Vamik Volkan (1995), who introduced the idea of the "seeds of madness": genuine "seeds" that, depending on developmental and relational vicissitudes, may remain silent or evolve into more severe psychopathological structures, such as psychotic or borderline conditions.

According to Volkan, such nuclei are formed in response to traumatic experiences, failures in developmental processes, and pathological interactions with primary caregivers. To defend himself from intolerable pain, the child develops mechanisms such as splitting, projection, and projective identification. Over time, as these mechanisms become rigidified, they form the basis of a psychotic or borderline mode of functioning.

Volkan underscores the importance of early relationships with caregivers: when they are inconsistent, intrusive, or excessively enmeshed, the child may internalize a disturbed image of both self and other. The seeds of madness do not merely represent traumatic experiences but psychic structures that shape the perception of reality and the way the individual relates to the world. Although initially latent, they may be reactivated by stressful events or specific relational dynamics, giving rise to psychotic symptoms or severe personality disorders. The result is a mode of functioning that privileges the sensory dimension over the symbolic one.

Volkan's concept proves particularly useful in understanding how some psychotic patients do not merely manifest a primitive mode of functioning, but rather have developed a pathological structure that privileges the sensory register at the expense of psychic elaboration. Although Volkan does not explicitly address the theme of infantile retreat, his conceptualization of the psychopathological evolution leading to psychosis strongly suggests the existence of an early withdrawal, originating in distorted emotional communication, if not in the intrusiveness of the primary objects into the child's mind.

These patients persistently live within a state of projective identification that takes them out of the world. Consequently, their introjective functions—essential for personal growth and the assimilation of experience—are gravely impaired. This limitation is reflected in the analytic process as well, explaining why such patients are often slow to grasp the insights offered by the analyst.

Living in a world dominated by concrete projective fantasies impoverishes both their vitality and their relational life. As a result, such patients appear passive and incapable of realistically planning their existence.

In the more advanced stages of the analytic process, it becomes possible to identify the infantile determinants that set the psychotic development in motion and to reconstruct the early conditions that established the subject's vulnerability to illness. It becomes evident that the withdrawal from reality had begun long before the clinical manifestations became apparent.

The analytic treatment of such patients requires an in-depth knowledge of the primary processes—namely, the child's distorted relations with his objects—which, from the outset, alter the developmental space and give rise to mental transformations whose consequences are often difficult to reverse.

Within the analytic encounter, it is essential to engage with those parts of the self that have remained outside the psychotic system, a task that tends to become less arduous in the later phases of the treatment when these develop more. The psychotic solution, in fact, exerts a powerful attraction upon the healthy part of the personality, and since the psychotic world functions as an exhilarating psychic resource for the patient, it is understandable that he defends it tenaciously and mistrusts the analyst.

Chapter 11

Psychosis and Destructiveness

As I have already noted several times, Bion, in his early phase, focused on psychosis by following the path indicated by Melanie Klein, who had emphasized the expelling function of projective identification as a typical feature of the schizoid–paranoid position.

In "On Identification" (1955), however, Klein broadens the perspective: projective identification is not only a tool for expelling intolerable fragments of the self, but also a means of appropriating the most desirable and envied aspects of the other. This is what happens to Fabien, the protagonist of Julien Green's story, who employs this mechanism not only to rid himself of unwanted parts of himself, but above all to seize the qualities of others that he most admires. In this movement, Fabien alters his own identity and, with it, his perception of reality.

The attack on reality, then, does not arise solely from hatred of it, but also from the fraudulent pleasure of possessing what belongs to the other.

If we consider this second meaning of projective identification, we understand how the distortion of reality stems from a dynamic of appropriation of desired qualities—success, power, pleasure—grounded in a narcissistic and omnipotent ideal of the self.

When Klein describes Fabien's incessant identifications, she underlines the manner in which the psychotic part of the personality eventually subjugates the entire personality, making it exceedingly difficult to escape its dominion.

Bion's initial model does not fully follow this path, but remains tied to his first conception of projective identification as an expulsive movement, typical of the schizoid–paranoid position. From this perspective, psychosis appears primarily as the bearer of destructive, dissociative, and separating actions.

In his writings, this refrain recurs with force, but at the expense of a richer description of the deceptions and sophisticated maneuvers through which the psychotic part conquers the patient. At times it seems that Bion reduces the illness itself to the destructive violence of the psychotic part and its hatred of reality.

This does not mean that he loses sight of the heart of the process, since the patient's personal identity is nonetheless annulled. However, his emphasis on

DOI: 10.4324/9781003765363-12

destructive action risks impoverishing the clinical picture, overshadowing the seductive dimension through which the psychotic part exercises its power.

In psychotic transformation, in fact, it is not only the frontal attack that is at work, but also the beguiling promise of a new identity: the illusion of abandoning one's real self in order to assume a different one, capable of guaranteeing a kind of psychic beatitude. It is enough to alter the perception of reality and surrender to the ecstasy of hallucination to convince oneself that this promise is authentic.

The allure of a world generated by the omnipotence of fantasy exerts a powerful seduction. By surrendering to extraordinary psychic experiences, the psychotic patient enters a mental universe that, step by step, slips out of his control: shipwreck comes after a voyage lived without regret, but it carries with it the anguish of an irreversible loss and of an impossible return.

Psychosis can be imagined as the exchange of a small but authentic patrimony for a pile of counterfeit banknotes: in the illusion of possessing wealth and power, the subject realizes—too late—that he has lost what was real. What remains is only the counterfeit money, while the original patrimony is no longer recoverable. This is the dilemma that the patient faces along his path.

The Healthy Part

In his early works, Bion sought to repair the patient's split ego, attempting to lead him back along the path that had brought him to fragmentation. Even after clearly distinguishing the psychotic part from the healthy part of the personality, however, he does not describe the ways in which the psychotic part conquers and subjugates the healthy one; rather, he insists on its hatred for reality and for those psychic functions that make awareness possible. In this way, the psychotic part appears as a purely destructive mental state: a voracious, envious, and cruel force that annihilates every attempt at reconstruction. The therapeutic space seems to close before an unrelenting violence.

Although Bion acknowledged the existence of a healthy part, he did not attribute to it an active function in the work of repair: he remained focused on the excessive aggressiveness expressed through projective identification. His attention was directed toward the need to recompose the fragmented ego, without considering that it might be precisely the healthy part of the personality that could serve as the nucleus capable of containing and transforming the psychotic part.

Thus, he did not follow Abraham's suggestion to work, with severely ill patients, in the "free intervals": that is, in the case of the psychotic patient, to patiently cultivate a space in which the analyst might engage in dialogue with the healthy part—even if minimal—and make it the fulcrum of the treatment.

In my view, the task that Bion left unfinished finds an essential continuation in the work of Rosenfeld. What is striking is how, in modifying his approach, Rosenfeld gradually abandoned the idea that psychotic patients could be treated within the same framework as neurotics. I personally consider this intuition fundamental: psychotic transference is not merely a phenomenon to be analyzed, but a potentially dangerous event capable of undermining the entire therapeutic process.

I believe Rosenfeld grasped with great clarity the value of Bion's concept of the psychotic part and the healthy part. It is within this polarity that the destiny of the cure is played out: when the psychotic part prevails, transference is transformed into a delusional field that draws the analyst into its vortex. For this reason, I share Rosenfeld's insistence on the need to show the patient how the psychotic part seduces, deceives, and distorts his judgment of reality.

It seems to me that Rosenfeld here takes up the intuition already anticipated by Bion, although too fleetingly, in his theory of projective transformations: what matters is not only to interpret, but to help the patient perceive how objective reality is manipulated and distorted. In this light, delusion no longer appears merely as destruction or hatred of reality, but as the creation of an illusory world of absolute pleasure, a seductive elsewhere that renders awareness powerless.

I fully endorse Rosenfeld's emphasis: the psychotic part is not static, a sort of pole in equilibrium with the rest of the personality, but a living force endowed with invasive power, capable at any moment of colonizing and engulfing the healthy part. It is precisely in this dynamic and dangerous conception of the psychotic part that I see the most original and fruitful advancement of his thought.

Bion himself had already intuited this mechanism when he wrote that the distance between the psychotic and the healthy part tends progressively to widen, to the point of rendering any mutual relationship impossible. In my view, this is the key: psychosis does not merely generate fragmentation, but digs an abyss that prevents any internal dialogue, leaving the subject imprisoned within a single mental register.

Psychotic Confusion

One must add a common problem in the psychotic state: the confusion between the healthy and the psychotic parts of the mind. The psychotic part offers the patient a pleasurable, sensually rewarding reality, making it appear not only useful but even essential for psychological survival. Consequently, the patient protects and conceals the delusion from the therapist, since he regards the psychotic part as healthy, insofar as it is a source of pleasure.

Bion himself, after all, had grasped the fascination of this dissociated world: it attracts precisely because it promises an existence without limits, free from the frustrations imposed by reality.

It is a world that seduces with its illusion of absolute freedom. In my view, it is in this light that the attack on linking should be read: not so much as a purely destructive act, but as an attempt to realize a dream of total liberation.

To construct such a universe, the patient must manipulate his sensory organs and suspend the very capacity to think. Yet, because this process is often accompanied by a pleasurable state, he does not perceive its peril. I believe this is where the most dangerous trap lies: in the illusion of opening himself to an unlimited space, the subject in fact builds a prison from which it will be later almost impossible to escape.

Bion states this without ambiguity: the patient cannot free himself from his psychotic prison, because he has destroyed the very instruments that would have allowed him to do so. The more the withdrawal engulfs psychic life, the more concrete the risk of irreversible absorption into psychosis becomes. Here, in my view, we touch upon the clinical core of the issue: a mind compelled to produce sensations and images without limit—an outcome of the inversion of the alpha function—does not generate thought, but an unstoppable flood of delusions and hallucinations.

To illustrate more clearly the relationship between the psychotic and non-psychotic parts of the personality—and, in particular, the attractive and seductive pull that the former exerts upon the latter—I would like to present two clinical examples. These are two dreams brought into session by two different patients, yet they share significant common elements. Both dreams are meaningful because they allow us to reconstruct the patient's active participation in the construction of the psychotic state.

Claudio is a young patient who has experienced an episode of grandiosity, followed by a persecutory delusion that continues to surface in his analysis. Here is one of his particularly relevant dreams:

> I am in a dark tunnel, like an underground station, and I try to reach the open air by climbing a staircase that leads upward. The staircase is extremely long and fantastical, like something out of a Miró painting. As I climb, I meet a man holding a sign that says: "These last five minutes will be the most terrible of your life."

In the dream, the persecutory scenario—which faithfully reproduces the persecution of his waking life—acquires a new meaning precisely because it is dreamed: the patient becomes a coauthor of the danger that threatens him. The dream scene thus reveals not only Claudio's passivity in the face of persecution, but also his unconscious intentionality in constructing the delusion.

The second dream belongs to Ada, a patient who had undergone an episode of delusional excitement followed by hospitalization, and who later began analytic treatment:

> I'm at a Dalí exhibition. There is an empty antechamber with columns resembling the giraffe-necks of the women painted by Dalí. I ask Dalí to accompany me into a room because I'm afraid. He takes me somewhere else and makes me eat a piece of a Madonna sculpture where the words

> "It's already too late" are written. I ask him to take me home because I don't have my car keys. The car turns into a treadmill; you climb it by pulling an elastic band with your hands. It's very steep, I laugh like a madwoman and fall backwards.

Ada associates the dream with her attraction to Dalí's work and to surrealism, with automatic writing that "frees the unconscious," and with the mental logorrhea that had led to her hospitalization. She recounts that, in the past, she had periods of graphomania in which she wrote for days without stopping. These were moments when her mind generated endless connections, an incessant and lucid flow of thought accompanied by an intense sense of exaltation.

In both dreams—though they belong to different patients—similar elements appear, among them the presence of surrealist painters who fascinate them because of their ability to transform reality. The two artists clearly represent the psychotic part of the personality: a part that initially seduces the mind with promises of freedom and imaginative power, and then, once it has captured the healthy part, overwhelms it and leads it into a state of psychic terror.

It becomes evident that both patients idealize the mad part of the personality, experiencing it as exciting and vital. Interpreting the dream as propaganda of the delusional part—and describing its seductive power—enables the analyst to show the patient that it is precisely a part of the self that creates, and believes in, the delusion.

These two dreams are not symbolic dreams in the classical sense; they correspond instead to *delusional dreams*, in which the delusional content is not disguised but shown in its very unfolding. Although different in theme—persecutory for Claudio, manic for Ada—they clearly illustrate the dynamic relationship between the psychotic and the healthy parts of the personality.

A Relational Perspective

In Bion's first phase, closer to Melanie Klein, the constitutional perspective prevails. The psychotic part of the personality appears as a destructive mental state present from birth, fueled by the death drive *and* sustained by pride and arrogance. It is this matrix that, in the psychotic patient, leads to the attack on linking, to envy and arrogance—forces that shatter the possibility of a convivial encounter with the object, barring access to the world of symbols and emotions.

Over time, however, a second perspective emerges, which I consider particularly fertile: the relational one. Here the focus shifts to the defect of the container, to the failed introjection of essential functions for affective symbolization. The psychotic part finds nourishment not only in its original destructive force, but also in maternal deficiency: the absence of an intuitive function capable of receiving the child's projective identification. In the absence of such receptivity, infantile communication is devalued and stripped of meaning, and the child is left alone to bear unbearable anxieties, eventually collapsing into *nameless dread*.

In my view, it is precisely in the tension between these two poles—the original drive and the relational wound—that the most authentic core of Bion's thought on psychosis may be discerned.

Yet one striking point in Bion's work on psychosis is his choice to almost completely disregard the patient's individual history: we find no references to childhood experiences, nor to the occasional circumstances that may have triggered the psychotic episode. His intuitions seem to emerge from an observational vertex that illuminates the elements of an impersonal process, as if psychosis were a movement of the universal mind rather than the particular story of a single individual.

This approach becomes evident in his description of the transformation into hallucinatory states. Bion analyzes it through a lens that could be called geometric–epistemological, attentive to grasping its logical and formal structures rather than its biographical and psychodynamic contents.

In my view, it is as if Bion left open the possibility that hallucinatory transformation could emerge in anyone: an eventuality inscribed within the potentiality of the human mind, not merely the outcome of a particular personal history. In this way, psychosis is conceived as a structural risk active in every individual.

When emotional input from the caregiver is lacking, the child uses his own body as an instrument of excitation. This outcome already constitutes the beginning of a transformation into hallucinatory states. Various forms of withdrawal can become the means by which to create sensory, sexualized, grandiose, and persecutory worlds, permeated with omnipotence.

In these cases, instead of developing thought and nourishing psychic reality, the mind is employed as a sensory organ, which, in the advanced stage of the psychotic process, leads to hallucinatory production. This possibility is already implicit in Bion's conceptualization, when he hypothesized that, parallel to thought (whose development he charted in the grid), a delusional system might also develop (described in his negative grid).

Chapter 12

Convergences and Divergences

The revolution introduced by Bion through his theory of the mind opened entirely new horizons: on the one hand, it enabled a deeper understanding of the psychotic state; on the other, it was his observation of psychosis that allowed him to elaborate a new theory of thinking.

The starting point is at once simple and radical: consciousness of reality exists, but it may be obliterated or cancelled. This divarication is what distinguishes neurotic from psychotic functioning. In the psychotic subject, projective identification acquires an omnipotent quality, capable of paralyzing the psychic apparatus. It is this mechanism that makes possible the withdrawal from reality.

This constitutes an essential divergence: the neurotic part works through assimilation, introjection, discrimination; the psychotic part, by contrast, proceeds through violent projections, impelled by the need to evacuate those psychic elements that the mind cannot "digest." Neurosis represses; psychosis expels.

Within this evacuative logic, the psychotic mind functions as a machine of expulsion: it casts out frustrating objects, experienced as bad, thus momentarily freeing itself from tension—but at the price of a radical impoverishment of psychic life.

I would now like to linger on some crucial points in Bion's intuitions and to ask to what extent they remain clinically fertile today, or whether they have remained confined to the theoretical plane.

It is certain that without Bion and Rosenfeld we would not possess a true psychoanalytic theory of psychosis. In particular, through his theory of thinking and his distinction between the healthy and psychotic parts of the personality, Bion opened a dynamic perspective: psychosis no longer appears as a regression to primitive developmental stages, but rather as the expression of an impaired capacity to think—a defect in the functions that transform sensory perceptions into thoughts.

In this light, the patient is not so much imprisoned in an irremediable primitiveness as in an incapacity to elaborate symbolically and to attribute meaning to the events of his psychic life. This is a model I find extraordinarily

DOI: 10.4324/9781003765363-13

contemporary, one that rescues psychosis from reductive readings and acknowledges its specific dramatic nature.

And yet, one cannot but observe that Bion's most visionary intuitions still fascinate us, but have found little operative translation on the clinical level. Bion remains revered as a great theorist of the mind, but his influence is not palpable when one descends to the concrete level of analytic work with psychotic patients.

It remains true, however, that it was precisely the mystery of psychosis that impelled him to investigate the origins of thought, and in this sense his reflection remains an indispensable legacy. It therefore seems useful, at this point, to gather and arrange Bion's contributions that still retain decisive value for clarifying the nature of the psychotic process.

1) Projective Identification

The first point to emphasize is the central role of projective identification. Much of the psychotic universe is constructed through this mechanism, capable of transforming the patient's identity to the point of severing every bond with reality and with the self. It is a genuine psychic metamorphosis, an extreme "projective transformation," as Bion conceived it, in which nothing remains stable or invariant.

This distortion of the perception of self and others corresponds to what Melanie Klein had glimpsed in the novel whose protagonist is Fabien (1955): through projective identification, the patient not only expels unwanted parts of himself but also merges with idealized and omnipotent figures, often characters of fantasy. In this way he assumes magical or terrifying qualities, remaining trapped in an identity that does not belong to him, without perceiving the loss of his inner reality.

In my view, Bion pushes this intuition beyond Klein's limits, describing a projective identification that is not merely seductive or illusory, but intrinsically destructive: a mechanism that devours from within the very possibility of self-recognition and of returning to oneself.

The patient's mind resorts to such a pervasive and intense use of projective identification that it cannot free itself from the identity into which it has been projected. This impossibility prevents him from recovering his own identity, entrapping him in a cycle of psychic confusion and capture.

Bion repeatedly emphasized in his clinical writings that massive use of projective identification inevitably entails a destructuring of time and space. It is particularly significant that this intuition, developed within his thought, finds an echo in other authors who, though proceeding from different premises, described the same phenomenon in other conceptual languages.

I am thinking of Federn's (1952) concept of *ego boundaries*. He conceived psychosis as a "disease of the ego," characterized by the inability to maintain the necessary boundaries and continuity of the ego. According to Federn, ego boundaries tend to dissolve because of the excessive presence of false ideas, which alter the perception of personal identity. This intuition proves extremely useful when related to Bion's concept of the healthy and psychotic parts of the personality.

It is evident that the psychotic part, operating through massive projective identifications, expands the ego into a dissociated world and dismantles the ego boundary—that mental and physical space within which our mind can operate. Only the healthy part, through the container function, is able to withstand and contain the devastating action of the psychotic part.

If psychosis originates in an infantile psychic retreat—a self-created world of dissociated and intensely sensory fantasies—then such a non-communicative realm develops without a container capable of receiving and integrating these experiences. In essence, the psychotic mind may be conceived as a *mind without a container*: the psychotic process unfolds precisely because there is no mental container able to receive and organize psychic experience.

When Bion introduces his conception of projective identification for communicative purposes, he underlines an important reversal: the negative aspects are displaced onto the person caring for the patient. In this perspective, the destructive attacks—rooted in early privations—appear to originate not so much from the patient as from the analyst himself.

Hatred, then, does not arise from a purely destructive drive, and the analyst is not the target of the patient's aggressiveness; he becomes rather the figure of that primary object that denied the very possibility of communication.

Here lies, in my opinion, one of Bion's most precious warnings: the analyst must learn to recognize the patient's language and to offer him the experience that a channel of communication truly exists. If this does not occur, the risk is that the analytic relationship turns into an impasse, a transference psychosis where the failure of communication is repeated and crystallized in the figure of the analyst as a bad object, a persecutor.

Bion's concept of projective identification as a communicative function—highlighting the role of the mother as a container of the child's verbal and non-verbal communications, transforming them into thinkable experiences—proved crucial for contemporary psychoanalytic theory and clinical practice. Yet Klein's conceptualization (1946, 1955) of the massive use of projective identification, in its original meaning, remains, in my view, profoundly valuable for understanding the specific nature of the psychotic process.

When a patient becomes trapped entirely in the projective identification, he loses access to the apparatus of reality-testing—the very mechanism that could assist in reconstructing an authentic identity and a sense of reality, both of which are entirely lost and appear irretrievable.

2) Projective Transformation

Another highly important concept in Bion is that of projective transformation. As I have already said, whereas in neurosis the repressed truth continues to maintain a correspondence with conscious belief, in psychosis distortion eliminates any possibility of correspondence between the original reality and its transformation. It is a *hyperbolic transformation*, a radical process that erases every link between the original object and its transformed version (Bion, 1965).

In other words, psychosis is one of the ways in which the mind deceives itself, rendering it impossible to comprehend or reverse the process. On this point, however, Bion formulates an essential statement: the analyst's task is to accompany the patient backwards, that is, to share with him the path traversed during the course of transformation.

In my view, with a delusional patient this passage is inevitable and necessary: whenever the action of the psychotic part is analyzed, the analyst must accompany him in the search for the origin of the delusion, the conflict, the wound, or the frustration that generated it and help him identify the delusional path he has taken.

This holds true both for the first episode and for those that repeat themselves over the course of treatment. The analytic task thus becomes one of deconstructing the delusional experience, stripping it of its hyperbolic character, and restoring to it the kernel of truth it contains.

It is Bion himself who reminds us that truth nourishes the mind as food nourishes the body, whereas lies poison it and lead it to starvation. Without truth, the mind risks withering away and delusion corresponds to the construction of a big lie.

3) The Psychotic and Non-Psychotic Parts of the Personality

After Freud, we owe to authors such as Katan and Bion intuitions that remain of great relevance, particularly the distinction between the psychotic and neurotic parts of the personality.

I have already said that I use the term *psychotic part* somewhat differently from Bion, who defined it as that part of the personality dominated by destructive instincts, by hatred for internal and external reality, and fuelled by an excessive congenital predisposition to aggressiveness and envy.

In my view, the psychotic part is not rooted in destructiveness, but rather identifies with that aspect of the personality—active since childhood—capable of constructing a world that replaces and annuls human relational reality.

In fact, the manipulation of the organs of psychic perception can extend to extreme levels, to the point of creating special worlds in which the patient remains trapped—for example, states of sexualized well-being, perverse pleasure, or delusional psychic reality.

An illuminating example is offered by the analysis of Mildred, narrated by Rosenfeld in his volume *Psychotic States* (1965). Mildred was imprisoned in a fantasy that prevented her from relying on the analytic work. Within it, a devil took shape, attacking the good and righteous, binding and gagging them. If they managed to free themselves even for a breath, the devil immediately tightened the chains even more. The victims thus remained suspended in a liminal state, neither fully alive nor entirely dead, and resistance to the devil appeared futile, since he possessed absolute power.

Rosenfeld discerned in this fantasy the echo of a negative therapeutic reaction. In the play of transference, the analyst became the devil himself, the figure of the evil father. Yet such an interpretation ended up fuelling Mildred's suspicion and distress: she began to believe that the analyst was attempting to manipulate her mind and to penetrate it with violence.

Before Bion's conceptualization, the psychotic part was not clearly identified as a phenomenon in its own right, as in the case of Rosenfeld, but was often interpreted through the lens of transference.

In this early phase of his work with psychotic patients, Rosenfeld did not perceive the devil fantasy as an internal object, a pathological structure, or a psychotic part of the personality aimed at dominating and alienating the patient from therapy. He interpreted it rather as a transferential expression of a sadistic paternal figure.

At the time of Rosenfeld's writings, indeed, Bion's concept of the psychotic part of the personality had not yet been formulated.

I believe that the concept of the psychotic part of the personality—understood as a psychopathological organization that dominates the rest of the personality—is not only useful for a psychodynamic understanding of the psychotic process, but also represents the keystone for entering a therapeutic dimension with the patient.

In my view, the core of our analytic work with psychotic patients consists in creating a triangulation founded on the dialogue between two non-psychotic minds—the non-psychotic part of the patient's mind and the analyst's mind—that collaborate to analyze the third vertex of the triangle: the patient's psychotic part. This triangle has a double function.

On the one hand, it allows for the identification of the psychotic part of the personality—capable of fascinating or terrifying the patient—and opens a dialogue with the healthy part in order to contain and transform the psychotic element, gradually reducing its power. On the other hand, it stimulates the growth of the patient's healthy personality, progressively making him more capable of entering into contact with the sphere of emotions, interpersonal relations, and the real world. In this process, the analyst assumes the role of a new object, helping the patient to develop experiences that had been precluded to him by the absence of an adequate internal and external container, originally provided by the parental figures.

Naturally, an authentic dialogue is not possible from the outset. The psychotic patient does not experience his psychotic part as mad or dangerous; on the contrary, he tends to idealize it, to regard it as the healthiest part, since it provides him with pleasure, power, and a sense of superiority. The analyst is often perceived with suspicion, as one who would deprive him of that source of strength. As I already said, for this reason, patients jealously guard their secret world, hidden in psychosis, avoiding any sharing of it.

It then becomes the task of the therapist's sensitivity to intuit, even before the patient communicates it, the presence of this world, to open a breach into it, and to attempt, with delicacy, to share it with the patient. In this regard, certain psychotic dreams—through which the delusional structure transparently reveals itself—may become clinical tools of great value.

The work to establish contact with the patient, however, demands time: months, at times years. The analyst must exercise patient waiting, moving with caution, yet without falling either into passivity or into collusion with the patient's delusional propaganda.

4) Attack on Linking

The hypothesis of an original destructiveness in the psychotic—endorsed by the Kleinian group—has found wide resonance in psychoanalytic discourse. It explains how the relationship with the world is marked by splitting and fragmentation: unable to tolerate the object as a source of creativity, the patient attacks it out of envy, simultaneously striking his own perceptual ego, which disintegrates and produces bizarre objects.

According to this conceptualization, the psychotic part is characterized by an incapacity to tolerate frustration and by the absence of the object. This intolerance to frustration is closely tied to excessive envy, which Bion identified as a central factor in psychotic functioning, particularly in early infancy.

Excessive envy leads to a profound hatred of any relational bond. This manifests as an attack on the link, a destructive process that undermines the capacity for symbolic thought and the formation of meaning. By destroying the symbolic language necessary to establish connections between experiences, such an attack renders the psychotic mind incapable of understanding and interpreting reality.

The conceptualization of the attack on linking is undoubtedly suggestive and bears witness to Bion's extraordinary creativity in the face of phenomena that seem to resist any explanation. Yet, as I have already observed, the hypothesis of an original destructiveness in psychosis appears to me the most questionable point of his early theory. Not by chance, in the second phase of his work Bion no longer mentions it, a sign that his thought had taken a different direction.

In my view, it is not necessary to postulate a systematic attack on the link to account for the splitting, fragmentation, and psychic catastrophe we observe in psychosis.

Rereading *Cogitations* (1992), which gathers precious fragments of Bion's thought, one encounters several reflections on the origin of psychosis. According to the author, when the infant experiences rage, he is confronted with death wishes: he would like the object to disappear, to be dead or non-existent.

The relationship with a living, vital object corresponds to alpha-elements; the dead, the link with an inert object to beta-elements. In the very first moments of existence, the infant is entirely dominated by the pleasure principle: where he feels satisfaction, he experiences himself surrounded by proto-real objects perceived as alive and present. But as soon as pain appears, the inner scene changes radically: the infant's hatred destroys the objects, transforming them into dead or non-existent ones.

When intolerance of frustration becomes more pronounced, what is attacked is not only the object but the very apparatus destined to transform sensory impressions into material suitable for thought. This destruction contributes to the sensation that it is "things," not words or ideas, that inhabit the personality.

The flight into psychosis—with all its destructive maneuvers—is thus an attempt to escape pain and frustration. However, Bion leaves unresolved the crucial question: why do some individuals, despite difficulties, pain, and frustration, manage to grow, while others enter into the psychotic illness?

In fact, we return to the problem I have already raised in this text. If one neglects the influence of the environment—that is, the mind of the caregiver—then one can only respond, as Melanie Klein did, that it is the child's aggressive charge that will determine his destiny.

If instead we take up what Bion himself emphasized, albeit mainly on a theoretical level, and place the accent on the importance of the child's communicative projective identification and the necessary empathic response of the maternal mind, then it will be the character of the latter that contributes to the child's choice between accepting emotional reality or, conversely, fleeing from it.

We must not forget that, in psychoanalytic observation, we do not only encounter parents who are insufficient or only partially adequate to foster the child's growth, but often parents who are clearly disturbed and possess active psychotic nuclei. What then becomes of the child's mind, seduced or frightened by the intrusions coming precisely from those who should care for him? What healthy identifications will in fact be possible for him?

Bion underscores how intolerance of frustration and the omnipotent illusion of absolute freedom propel the subject toward boundless spaces. Yet this expansion does not translate into genuine freedom: it culminates rather in an explosion that delivers the subject into a boundless panic.

In their inner worlds, these patients aspire to create a mental space detached from the laws of relation and thought, a territory imagined as free from bonds, devoid of temporal and spatial limits. In this alternative universe they imagine themselves as absolute masters of their own mind, which proceeds without contradictions, as if everything were possible.

This is what I consider a psychic withdrawal: the place where thoughts are replaced by sensory representations that flow without rules or logic, assuming the value of revelations. Psychic reality yields to sensory reality: it is not so much an attack on thought as a substitution of thought with processes of a perceptual nature. But to remain too long in this space means losing the way back: the patient no longer knows how to use the mind as an instrument of thought that is definitively erased. The two worlds, sensory and psychic, cannot coexist; one erases the other.

For this reason, as Bion repeatedly observes, in the psychotic we find no traces of *reverie* nor alpha-elements, and therefore none of the functions that depend on them: attention, capacity for judgment, creative imagination.

The mind in psychotic state organizes itself differently: it may function as a sensory organ rather than as an apparatus of thought. It makes use of images, auditory perceptions, bodily experiences, which construct a narrative lived as real. In this way, over the years, states of sensory confusion are structured that precipitate into recurrent psychotic crises.

The continuous use of the mind as a purely perceptual organ corrodes the possibility of thought and, paradoxically, denies the patient precisely that freedom he was pursuing. For, by destroying the instruments that would have permitted a return to psychic reality, he condemns himself to an existence imprisoned in a sensory world—unlimited, yet sterile.

We cannot overlook the indispensable contribution of Wilfred Bion's creative work on the theory of thinking for understanding some fundamental nodes of the psychotic process, among them the phenomenon I have described as *infantile sensory retreat*. Bion's reflections offer a conceptual framework that allows us to approach those forms of psychic functioning in which thinking fails to develop as a transformative activity applied to sensory experience.

Particularly illuminating in this regard is the concept of the *container–contained* relationship. As already suggested, the psychotic patient's thoughts lack an adequate container capable of making them thinkable. They are thoughts that do not encounter a mind able to receive, hold, and transform them. In Bion's well-known formulation, they may therefore be described as thoughts without a thinker.

The hypothesis of infantile sensory retreat as an initial moment in psychotic development helps us understand how a mode of psychic functioning may arise that proceeds, at least in part, in the absence of a container capable of transforming sensory experience. Within the Bionian model, symbolization emerges precisely from the encounter between container and contained: the child's primitive emotional experiences, initially unthinkable, can become thoughts only insofar as they meet a mind capable of receiving them and transforming them within a symbolic register.

This function is originally performed by the maternal mind through that particular capacity Bion called *reverie*. By receiving the infant's raw emotional states—what Bion described as beta-elements—the mother transforms them through the alpha function into elements that can be thought. She then returns them to the infant as experiences endowed with meaning. In this way, the infant gradually acquires the capacity to think his or her own emotional states.

In the course of normal development, the infant therefore remains in a structuring dependence upon the maternal mind. This dependence concerns not only physical survival but constitutes the very condition for the emergence of the capacity to think and to experience emotions as meaningful. Through the relationship with the other's mind, the child gradually learns to participate in the construction of a *shared symbolic world*.

In infantile retreat by contrast, a part of the psyche withdraws from this structuring dependence that is essential for mental development. The infant's container—represented by the parents' thinking—becomes, in withdrawal, obscured and unavailable, failing to be internalized as a function of the self.

What comes into being, then, is a *separate psychic domain*, predominantly sensory in nature. This self-sufficient world, grounded in immediate sensoriality rather than symbolic transformation, allows the individual to evade both the developmental demands of mental growth and the pressures of shared reality.

It is precisely this possibility of a psychic functioning partially autonomous from the transformative relationship with the other, brought into focus by Bion's theory of thinking, that helps illuminate certain essential aspects of psychotic development.

5) Interpretation

Psychotic patients, who operate predominantly at a sensory level, lack the mechanism of repression as well as the capacity to represent and symbolize. In other words, they do not possess an active dynamic unconscious and, consequently, cannot rely on intuition to understand themselves, nor are they able to generate dreams endowed with meaningful psychic content.

This difficulty highlights the divergence of approaches among different therapeutic models, particularly between Kleinian analysts (such as Rosenfeld, Segal, and Bion), who regard transference interpretations as both necessary and feasible, and other orientations that do not place interpretative work as a central point.

Among the latter, I would emphasize the contributions of Frieda Fromm-Reichmann and Paul Federn, whose insights, in my view, remain of great value for the therapeutic treatment of psychosis.

Fromm-Reichmann (1959) and Federn (1952), both of whom worked extensively with psychotic patients, agreed that the interpretative approach used with neurotic patients is not suitable for those suffering from psychosis. They argued that symbolic–analytic interpretations are not only ineffective but may in fact be misleading for psychotic patients, whose minds are overwhelmed by a continuous flood of sensory impressions and multiple, often contradictory, meanings.

Fromm-Reichmann, in particular, contended that the therapeutic approach with psychotic patients should not be based on traditional interpretation but rather on an attempt to understand how the delusional world invades the patient's mind. This implies a shift away from symbolic interpretation toward an examination of the very nature of the patient's internal experience.

Federn further emphasized that, in the case of a manifest psychotic state, the analyst's primary task is to share and accept the falsifications generated by the patient's delusion. This means that the therapist must enter the patient's delusional world, acknowledging it as part of his or her experience.

Only after establishing a relationship of trust can the analyst begin to address the delusional attitude—that is, the way in which the patient's mind distorts or even erases reality. According to Federn, symbolic interpretations, including those concerning transference, would only deepen the patient's confusion, since the psychotic ego is already highly fragmented.

For psychotic patients, whose minds are saturated with an excess of meanings, encouraging free associations—as is customary in the treatment of neurotics—is not advisable. On the contrary, their imagination should in some measure be contained, so as to prevent further chaos in their mental landscape.

A crucial point stressed by Federn is that psychotic patients cannot make use of repression in the same way as neurotic patients. As a result, their unconscious does not function dynamically. In other words, unlike neurotic patients who are able to relegate disturbing thoughts and feelings into the unconscious, psychotic patients lack this defensive mechanism to keep troubling or distressing material at a distance, thereby complicating their mental processes even further.

The Kleinian group developed a rich and complex theory of psychotic disorders, introducing such fundamental concepts as projective identification (Klein), symbolic equation (Segal), psychotic transference (Rosenfeld), the bizarre object, the attack on linking, and the psychotic part of the personality (Bion).

These ideas played a significant role in the understanding and treatment of psychosis from a Kleinian perspective. Nevertheless Kleinian analysts maintained that psychotic patients can be treated in a manner analogous to neurotic patients, employing techniques such as the analysis of transference, dreams, and communication. Rosenfeld, in the first part of his work, emphasized the importance of preserving these essential features of psychoanalysis even in the work with schizophrenia.

I believe that the failure to untie this fundamental knot in a clear and articulated way has contributed to diverting attention from the treatment of psychosis in recent decades—an interest that cannot be abandoned if psychoanalysis wishes to continue engaging with the unknown and with what still remains to be discovered.

Conclusions

In these pages, I have sought to retrace the path outlined by Bion in his exploration of psychosis, beginning with his earliest clinical writings. Like other authors—Rosenfeld comes to mind—he initially moved within the Kleinian framework, assuming that the understanding of psychotic processes required the coordinates delineated by Melanie Klein: projective identification, splitting, and the denial of reality.

Bion believed that by applying these concepts to clinical work, one could bring about an improvement in the patient's clinical constellation. Many years later, Rosenfeld would reflect on this initial framework and state: "A clearly defined method of approaching psychotic states is important if we expect to do research to clarify the psychotic psychopathology rather than concentrating on symptomatic improvement" (1969, p. 615). In simple terms: one cannot rush ahead under the illusion of "curing" the patient without first dwelling upon the mystery of psychosis itself.

To demonstrate how much the analyst must learn before embarking on this kind of therapy, Rosenfeld made a statement that may appear pessimistic, yet I find it realistic and profoundly useful.

He maintained (Rosenfeld, 1987) that analysts should learn *afresh* how to treat psychotic patients, since what they have learned in working with "normal" patients does not function in these cases. Analysts should even consider acquiring new therapeutic skills by undertaking specific training.

I believe this judgment to be sound, because once one enters the field of psychosis, the laws that regulate psychic activity in the neurotic world (repression, sublimation, conflict, censorship, etc.) no longer apply. The laws of unconscious thought discovered by psychoanalysis concern the functioning of psychic reality as it operates within the dynamic unconscious, which is not active in the psychotic state, where sensory reality prevails.

Indeed, the traditional analytic categories we are accustomed to employing—categories derived from the dynamic unconscious—do not enable us to grasp the specific nature of psychotic illness and the way in which it manifests itself in an apparently bizarre and enigmatic manner.

DOI: 10.4324/9781003765363-14

Only by relinquishing what we have learned during our training can we expand our knowledge and assist these patients in finding a path toward recovery. In other words, we must work like a physicist studying atoms, who does not rely on the laws of mechanical physics, knowing he is faced with a field of entirely different phenomena.

From this perspective, Bion has provided a body of knowledge of extraordinary importance. Today, this allows us to conceive of psychosis as a planet open to exploration, beginning with the function of thought—an indispensable instrument of life, which operates beyond conscious awareness and must take root firmly from the very earliest moments of existence, so that it does not disperse or fragment when confronted with knowledge and reality.

As analysts, and in a way akin to Freud—who initially regarded transference as an obstacle and later as an agent of change—we too must attend with utmost care to the emergence of psychotic functioning within analysis, with its continuous transformations and risks, as a normal occurrence of therapy and as the key to a possible resolution of the analytic process.

For this reason, I believe that future analytic inquiry must extend to the territories of the mind that have been only partially explored, namely those mental conditions—such as the psychotic state—that lie beyond the unconscious functioning we already know.

Those observations apply perfectly to Bion's trajectory. In the initial phase, he believed that the analyst's task consisted in facilitating, through interpretative work, the recomposition of the fragments of the patient's ego, progressively bringing together what was split and dispersed.

Yet, when faced with patients in an acute phase or enclosed for years within their psychotic retreat, Bion repeatedly took note that the connective tissue necessary for repair did not exist: the psychic matter was too fragmented to be "stitched" together by interpretative instruments.

Nevertheless, Bion never abandoned the endeavor. The second part of his work seems entirely devoted to an exploration and deepening that no longer moved solely from the Kleinian vertex. The problem of psychosis remained ever at the center of his thought. This is attested by the pages of *Cogitations*, scattered with annotations on psychosis, often written with the anguish of one who feels unable to find the key to an enigma that resisted any definitive clarification.

It is, however, from his theory of thinking that flashes emerge—intuitions of extraordinary fecundity, capable of illuminating the dark and arduous terrain of psychosis, and which have preserved their heuristic power. As with the great explorers, the destination is not always reached, but the outposts marked along the way remain indispensable for those who continue the journey.

Bion has left us signals, maps, and precious indications which, once integrated, allow us today to glimpse more clearly what for him remained in part unattainable. This is why his name, more than any other, remains bound to psychosis: to him we owe the merit of having opened new paths, shedding light upon a territory we still traverse with caution, but guided by roads that unmistakably bear his imprint.

At this point, a broad field opens for the future development of psychoanalytic inquiry into psychosis—its origins, its developmental course, and its treatment. The clinical task is to help the patient regain what has been lost, or what could not develop, during the earliest years of life—those formative moments in which the nucleus of personal identity, unique and unrepeatable in each individual, first takes shape.

Work must proceed along two lines. The first concerns helping the patient to move beyond a sensory mode of mental functioning, fostering the capacity for thinking. The second involves making possible the construction of an identity and a sense of self that have never been brought into being.

From this perspective, the psyche may be conceived as an entity structured according to unconscious organizing principles, formed in childhood within an intersubjective relational matrix. In this respect, Bion's contributions remain indispensable—his conceptualization of the alpha function, projective identification as a communicative process, and the container–contained relationship continue to offer a fundamental framework.

These complex and elusive psychic structures, grouped by Bion under the term *alpha function*, correspond to those mental operations situated at the level of the unconscious matrices of thought and emotion—processes inaccessible to language and beyond the reach of conscious understanding.

Bion stands as perhaps the most incisive explorer of this unknown territory (will we ever possess the means to truly know it?). In his theorization, the unconscious is reconceived as a psychic function that enables the mind to generate thoughts, though we lack the instruments to apprehend their origin and mode of construction.

Psychosis confronts us daily with the enigmatic processes of thought and psychic reality—a world that enables us to live, to know, and to learn, though all of this occurs largely outside awareness. There exists, indeed, an unconscious that comprehends the meaning of experience: an unknowing function of awareness itself—of external and internal reality, of the emotional field, and of the perception of body, space, and time. Yet even awareness may be lost.

In the psychotic transformation, awareness of what is occurring may be preserved for a time. During the initial phase of delusional experience, the patient may recover if he can rely on the healthy part of the self. Later, when self-awareness collapses, it becomes very difficult to come back; the patient ceases to experience alarm and yields passively to the advancing psychosis.

A crucial factor is the seduction exerted by the psychotic part upon the healthy one. When the patient constructs his world of sensory fantasies, he assumes the role of a god creating the universe and consequently becomes convinced of his superiority over other human beings—including the analyst. Under such conditions, it is evident that the patient lacks awareness and is unable to comprehend interpretations addressing his omnipotence.

It is difficult to describe with clarity the psychotic transformation—that moment when the spatio-temporal parameters organizing experience are abolished. Thoughts lose meaning, expanding to invade spaces that should remain neutral; events from the distant past reappear and are lived as though present; the mind undergoes limitless transformations. In psychotic thought, correspondences disintegrate, for everything unfolds under the sign of absolute omnipotence. Psychosis represents, in this sense, the transgressive manifestation *par excellence*, since the very rules of thinking are erased, allowing thought to proliferate at will—like a herd of wild horses set loose.

In this book devoted to Bion's thought, it was not possible to address the theme of psychosis in the broad and exhaustive terms it would have deserved. Since psychosis has been the focus of my research for several decades, the reader may refer to my other writings (De Masi, 2006, 2026). In this work, I have considered only those aspects that intersect with the path traced by Bion.

Keeping psychosis as a constant point of reference in his exploration of human thought is Bion's great merit. He followed an intuition of Freud, who wrote that only by studying the pathological do we come to understand the normal.

For this reason, psychosis constitutes a vast field of learning for psychoanalysts—a terrain from which much remains to be discovered.

References

Bion, W. (1954) Notes on the theory of schizophrenia. *The International Journal of Psychoanalysis*, 35, 113–118.

Bion, W. (1956) The development of schizophrenic thought. *The International Journal of Psychoanalysis*, 37, 344–346.

Bion, W. (1957) Differentiation of the psychotic from the non-psychotic personalities. *International Journal of Psychoanalysis*, 38, 266–275.

Bion, W. (1958) On hallucination. *International Journal of Psychoanalysis*, 39, 341–349.

Bion, W. (1959) Attacks on linking. *International Journal of Psychoanalysis*, 40, 308–315.

Bion, W. (1962a) *Learning from experience.* Routledge.

Bion W. (1962b) The psycho-analytic study of thinking. *International Journal of Psychoanalysis*, 43, 306–310.

Bion, W. (1965) *Transformations: Change from learning to growth.* Heinemann.

Bion, W. (1967) *Second thoughts.* Heinemann.

Bion. W. (1970) *Attention and interpretation: A scientific approach to insight in psychoanalysis and groups.* Tavistock Publications.

Bion, W. (1992) *Cogitations.* Estate of Wilfred R. Bion.

Bollas, C. (1987) *The shadow of object: Psychoanalysis of the unthought known.* Free Association.

Britton, R. (2015) *Mind and brain.* Karnac Books.

De Masi, F. (2006) *Vulnerability to psychosis: A psychoanalytic study of the nature and therapy of the psychotic state.* Karnac Books.

De Masi, F. (2020) *A psychoanalytic approach to treating psychosis: Genesis, psychopathology and case study.* Routledge.

De Masi, F. (2024) An enlightening concept: Psychic retreat, psychosis and other conditions. In H Weiss (Ed.), *The allure of psychic retreats: Clinical and theoretical inquiries. Celebrating the work of John Steiner.* Brandes & Apsel Verlag.

De Masi, F. (2025) *Beyond the dynamic unconscious.* Karnac.

De Masi, F. (2026) *Psychosis: A contemporary introduction.* Routledge.

Federn, P. (1952) *Ego psychology and psychosis.* Imago.

Freud, S. (1911) *Formulations on the two principles of mental functioning.* S. E. Vol.12.

Freud, S. (1924a) *Neurosis and psychosis.* S. E. Vol.19.

Freud, S. (1924b) *The loss of reality in neurosis and psychosis.* S. E. Vol.19.

Freud, S. (1938) *An outline of psychoanalysis.* S. E. Vol.23.

Fromm-Reichmann, F. (1959) *Psychoanalysis and psychotherapy: Selected papers of Frieda Fromm-Reichmann*. The University of Chicago Press.

Green, J. (1947) *Si j'etais vous*. E. Plon.

Grotstein, J. S. (1981) Who is the dreamer who dreams the dream and who is the dreamer who understands it? In *Do I dare disturb the universe?* Karnac Books.

Harris Williams, M. (2022) *Donald Meltzer: A contemporary introduction*. Routledge.

Katan, M. (1954) The importance of the nonpsychotic part of the personality in schizophrenia. *International Journal of Psychoanalysis*, 35(2), 119–128.

Klein, M. (1946) Notes on some schizoid mechanism. In *Envy and gratitude and other works, 1946–1963*. Hogarth.

Klein, M. (1955) On identification. In *Envy and gratitude and other works, 1946–1963* (pp. 31–50). Hogarth.

Meltzer, D. (1979) Un approccio psicoanalitico alla psicosi. *Quaderni di psicoterapia infantile. Le Psicosi*, 2, 31–50.

O'Shaughnessy, E. (1992) Psychosis: Not thinking in a bizarre world. In R. Anderson (Ed.), *Clinical lectures on Klein and Bion* (pp. 89–101). Tavistock.

Rosenfeld, H. (1950) Notes on the psychopathology of confusional states in chronic schizophrenia. *International Journal of Psychoanalysis*, 31, 132–137.

Rosenfeld, H. (1952) Notes on the psycho-analysis of the super-ego conflict of an acute schizophrenic patient. *International Journal of Psychoanalysis*, 33, 111–131.

Rosenfeld, H. (1965) *Psychotic states: A psychoanalytic approach*. Hogarth.

Rosenfeld, H. (1969) On the treatment of psychotic states by psychoanalysis: An historical approach. *International Journal of Psychoanalysis*, 50, 615–631.

Rosenfeld, H. (1971) A clinical approach to the psychoanalytic theory of the life and death instincts: An investigation into the aggressive aspects of narcissism. *International Journal of Psychoanalysis*, 52, 169–178.

Rosenfeld, H. (1987) *Impasse and interpretation*. The New Library of Psychoanalysis.

Segal, H. (1956) Depression in the schizophrenic. *International Journal of Psychoanalysis*, 37, 339–343.

Segal, H. (1957) Notes on symbol formation. *International Journal of Psychoanalysis*, 38, 391–397.

Steiner, J. (1993) *Psychic retreats: Pathological organizations of the personality in psychotic, neurotics and borderline patients*. Routledge.

Volkan, V. (1995) *The infantile psychotic self and its fates: Understanding and treating schizophrenics and other difficult patients*. Bloomsbury Academic.

Weiss, H. (Ed.) (2024) *The allure of psychic retreats: Clinical and theoretical inquiries. Celebrating the work of John Steiner*. Brandes & Apsel Verlag.

Index

For Product Safety Concerns and Information please contact our
EU representative GPSR@taylorandfrancis.com Taylor & Francis
Verlag GmbH, Kaufingerstraße 24, 80331 München, Germany